Dementia
New Skills for Social Workers

of related interest

Introducing Network Analysis in Social Work
Philip Seed
ISBN 1 85302 034 6 hb
ISBN 1 85302 106 7 pb

The Abuse of Elderly People
A Handbook for Professionals
Jacki Pritchard
Foreword by Professor Eric Sainsbury
ISBN 1 85302 122 9

Dementia
New Skills for Social Workers

Edited by Alan Chapman and Mary Marshall

Case Studies for Practice 5   General Editor: Philip Seed

Jessica Kingsley Publishers
London and Bristol, Pennsylvania

First published in the United Kingdom in 1993 by
Jessica Kingsley Publishers Ltd
116 Pentonville Road
London N1 9JB

Copyright © 1993 the contributors and the publisher

British Library Cataloguing in Publication Data
Chapman, Alan
Dementia: New Skills for Social Workers
– (Case Studies for Practice Series)
I. Title II. Marshall, Mary III. Series
362.2

ISBN 1 85302 142 3

Printed and Bound in Great Britain by
Biddles Ltd., Guildford and King's Lynn

Contents

Introduction

Mary Marshall

Working with people with dementia and their carers must be the most exciting field of social work to be in at the moment. What other field offers a dramatic increase in numbers making it a high priority for health, local authorities, private and voluntary agencies? What other field offers constantly changing approaches and constantly improving techniques? What other field offers a completely new area for social workers to use our well established skills (and make our name if we are minded to write about it)? What other area requires multidisciplinary work to such an extent that it challenges all the recent legislation and guidance on community care? What other field has new models of services being tried all the time? What other field is so free from protocol and procedure that imaginative practice is still really possible?

This is not to say that it is a field without intense frustrations and shortfalls. In spite of the increase in numbers, people with dementia and their carers are still not a political priority and new money is still poured into waiting list initiatives and life saving equipment. There is still a lot of poor if not bad practice. Many staff are woefully out of date in their skills and approach. Such is the rate of change that if you were trained more than five years ago you are likely to be out of date.

There is far too little emphasis on the need for the highest level of social work skills. In many places it is quite difficult to get any social work help since this work is channelled straight to unqualified staff. This will happen when social workers are more confident about what they have to offer – hence this book. We have opted to cover relatively obvious social work skills because we believe that it is in starting from what we know that we are most likely to develop our skills. We have also opted for people with something to say rather than simply covering the ground. Counselling was an obvious skill to include and we had a good contact in Iain Gardner who had run a counselling scheme for people with dementia and their carers in Melbourne. We turned again to Iain in our search for someone to write about family therapy since the two units we found in the UK providing family therapy to mentally ill older people had not worked much with people with dementia. He and his colleague have chosen to write a general paper on systemic work based on their experience of family therapy. No book on dementia would be complete without a chapter on the creative use of the past. We were fortunate that one of the major British experts, Faith Gibson, was willing to write for us.

Groupwork was another obvious skill that needs to be developed in this field and we have chosen to focus mainly on carers' groups since these are the most usual starting point. We have also chosen to have a chapter on empowerment because it is so important in a low status field such as this one. Care management was an obvious necessity and we were fortunate in having a local pilot project from which to learn. Finally, we needed to have something on network analysis for this series and we were very lucky that Philip Seed was willing to look at two real situations and to draw out the skill issues for us. This book is therefore clearly based in the land of the possible.

There is nothing too different about using our skills in this emerging field but it is rare to read about them or to hear social workers blowing their own trumpets.

One of the interesting dimensions we have been able to cover is multidisciplinary work: still far too rare in this field. Where it exists, for example in psychogeriatrics or primary health care, social work is invariably left out. The care management project presented here was actually a multidisciplinary one.

Finally, the very lack of protocol and procedure which can be so liberating can also reflect a lack of interest and poor practice. It may, for example, be better to use the Mental Health legislation more often since there is a lot of dubious practice which would not be contemplated with younger people. Locked doors for people who are not under section, for example, are illegal in the strict terms of the legislation. Few places have clear procedures to cover this kind of restraint. This illustrates the need for a great deal more social work practice and social work literature in this field.

CHAPTER ONE

New Trends and Dilemmas in Working with People with Dementia and their Carers

Mary Marshall

Why is it all so new and exciting? Fifteen years ago, when only a few enthusiasts such as the charismatic old age psychiatrists Drs Arie, Jolley, Pitt and Bergmann were proselytising and there were no social work books about dementia and the Winslow Press did not exist, it was generally assumed that people with dementia were totally unaware of their world. It was also assumed that carers were managing and if they were not their relative was in care, and that more of the service models of day hospital, home help and longstay care were what we needed to meet *The Rising Tide* (1982). The social workers in the teams that clustered round the rare but outstanding and committed psychiatrists were doing wonderful work but they were not the type of people to write up their practice. Pat Smith, a social worker, for example, who worked with Professor Jolley in the 1970s in Manchester was working with people with dementia in a way that would seem modern even today. She was prepared to enter the psychological reality of the person with dementia and to work with this to communicate and to offer choice. She was never persuaded to write up her practice to any extent.

Old fashioned practice assumes that dementia has a steady and predictable set of stages, that people with dementia are simply to be kept comfortable and their behaviour merely tolerated, and that carers do not wish to participate in care provided outside the home. It fails to listen to carers and undermines rather than empowers them. It is still widespread but it is increasingly recognised as unacceptable.

BASIC FACTS

This chapter deliberately did not begin with the usual facts and figures because these can be alarming and off-putting. We can all feel powerless and inadequate faced with the nature and extent of this tragic disease, but the purpose of this book is to engage and empower students and beginning social workers. It is nevertheless important to know the basics. These will be covered in a few paragraphs.

First, language; why do we use the term dementia rather than the somehow less frightening term, Alzheimer's disease? We use it because it is more accurate. In many ways we are at a point in dementia where we were with cancer 15 years ago. Then we referred to tumours or lumps. Sometimes we mentioned a highly specific kind of cancer such as a melanoma rather than use the awful 'C' word. Cancer is now widely talked about to the great comfort of many people with the disease or whose relatives have it. The same is true of dementia. Alzheimer's disease is only one sort of dementia, admittedly the main sort. About 50 per cent of the people with dementia have Alzheimer's disease. This is a global disease of the brain which progresses inexorably towards death, knocking out the functions of the brain as it goes. It starts with memory loss, as do most of the other dementias. About 20 per cent of people with dementia have multi-infarct dementia which is caused by strokes in the brain and has a rather less predictable course. Then there are a whole lot of other, relatively minor, diseases which cause dementia.

Dementia is not the same as confusion or delirium. Confusion is a symptom of both dementia and delirium and is not a diagnosis. It is one of those terms better not used because it is so easily misused, albeit often with kindly intent to avoid the real and painful word. It is in the category of 'lumps' instead of cancer. Delirium, or an acute confusional state as it is sometimes called, is caused by many things. Infections, bereavements, sudden changes and pain can cause delirium in any of us yet the symptoms are the same as dementia. The difference is that it usually comes on suddenly and that, properly identified, it can be treated. Depression is a complicating factor. It can cause delirium and it can exacerbate dementia. It can even be mistaken for dementia. Given that there is treatment for depression it is vitally important that it is recognised.

One in ten of us will get dementia and we will get it in old age. The older we are the more likely we are to get it. Nearly a million people in the UK have it already. There are several reasons why the numbers are increasing rapidly. The main one is that the baby bulge born at the turn of the century and before the Great War are now very old and from 65 onwards the proportion of people in each age group with dementia doubles every five years (Jorm and Korten 1986). Because of the population trends in the older population, the numbers of people with dementia will increase by 25 per cent between the years 1981 and 1996. There are also other groups emerging. People with Downs Syndrome are almost certain to get early onset dementia. Another emerging group is people with Aids. About 20 per cent of them get dementia. There are also a very small group of people who get early onset dementia, usually Alzheimer's but sometimes other forms such as Creutzfeldt-Jakob disease. The numbers of these people do not seem to be rising but they are increasingly recognised as a very needy group who do not fit into the services that, at present, exist.

Some text books list the *stages* of dementia. This can be useful but, like the concept of *stages of grief*, can be misleading. Dementia is a progressive disease that leads to death. It goes at different speeds for different people and everyone's pathway through the disease is unique. Usually there are seen to be three stages of progressive deterioration, the third being the terminal stage and it is useful to see it like this if it stops the generalising about the needs of people with dementia and their carers as a group. People with dementia and their carers will need different kinds of assistance at different stages. However, people will vary. Some people, for example, exhibit very troublesome behaviour quite early on, others later. Some remain sweet and pleasant throughout. Some people are very fit and energetic, other are very frail.

The commonly used labels: mild, moderate and severe are seldom enough. In themselves they do not tell you a great deal about the behaviour, personality and needs of a person with dementia. It is equally important to know whether or not they have any physical problems. It is, for example, essential to know if someone is able to walk or not or whether they have a hearing impairment. A good assessment of dependency across the board with information on physical needs, confusion, behaviour, and social skills is needed. Ongoing psychiatric disorder is another important kind of information. Are they suffering from depression or an anxiety state, for example? Finally, and every bit as important as the rest, what kind of person is this? Do they have a lot of unresolved business from the past, do they have good relationships, are they used to confronting problems or ignoring them and so on.

Having provided a brief resume of the basic information which every social worker should know, I want now to share what is new in this field.

Given the speed of change, this section on new skills, indeed the whole book, may soon be out of date, but the trends are becoming clearer. The changes in approach are partly the result of greater knowledge and experience, partly taking place as a result of the work of some very creative and imaginative professionals and partly due to the application of skills transferred from other client groups. This last is happening far too slowly. There are vast numbers of potentially helpful skills and approaches in other fields which could be tried. Perhaps the most fertile transfer would be from the field of learning disability where great strides have been made in small group living and the use of activities of daily living. But there are undoubtedly more skills to be drawn from child care and from the hospice movement.

CARERS

The real recognition of the contribution of carers has really only occurred in the last decade. At the macro level this is reflected in the increasing influence of carers' organisations; both the general ones such as The Carers' National Association and the specific ones which have grown out of self help groups such as the Alzheimer's Disease Society (or Alzheimer's Scotland). Their influence on politicians and policy makers is immense, albeit hard won. Carers have been written into the new community care legislation and policies from the beginning. There may be nasty hidden agendas about this in terms of making them carry a greater burden of (relatively cheap) care but even so their needs are now going to have to be acknowledged.

At the micro level, it would be an odd social worker who had not read anything about carers and the fundamental role they play in community care. They increasingly have a voice as a group, thanks to good back-up from their organisations. Most social workers will be, however dimly, aware of the stresses and strains of being a carer, and of their sacrifices: financial, social and personal. There are numerous books for carers and about carers. In this field the most significant is *The Thirty Six Hour Day* (Mace *et al.* 1985). Most policy documents have statements that talk about 'involving carers' although this can be a mere platitude as the lack of carer input to community care plans illustrates. Most social workers in this field would automatically be thinking about a carers' group, if not actually helping to run one.

What is missing is a real commitment to empowering carers. We also feel rather ambivalent about giving carers a voice, knowing that our service is not as good as we would like it to be. There is a chapter in this book on empowering, although the main discussion focuses on a training programme which aimed to empower carers.

Empowering requires a reframing of attitudes, although skills of advocacy, collaboration and partnership follow close behind.

Carers need to feel they are in control. For a carer the process of involving a professional in problems often means relinquishing control which can make them feel criticised by implication and thus diminished. Interventions can also lead to increasing guilt. The key, for the social worker, is active listening. Carers are often saying that they want to attend day care with their relative or want to assist in personal caring tasks, for example, but nobody hears because the carer does not know how to say it powerfully enough and because this is seldom what the providers want to hear. People seldom hear, at least the first time it is said, what they do not want to hear. Groups of carers are often run in a well meaning, but unformulated way by non-carers, once again making carers feel diminished. This is not to say that carers are, on the whole, unappreciative of the help they get both as individuals and as a group. Indeed they are usually pathetically grateful.

Applying groupwork knowledge to working with carers is also new. This is not to say that most carefully considered and sophisticated groups have not been run in the past for carers, but rather that these were not the norm. The more usual kind of group is vague in its purpose and makes little use of the skills and knowledge we all have, or should have, of basic groupwork. Carers' support groups play an important part in helping carers cope with the extremely varied and fluctuating emotions related to their burden of caring. However the agenda may be set by the professionals rather than the carers.

Alan Chapman, in a later chapter, contrasts 'traditional' support groups with a self help group and a therapeutic group. Significantly, the therapeutic group provided the opportunity for members to set an agenda and pursue outcomes which met their requirements. This is an area which seems ripe for development.

PEOPLE WITH DEMENTIA

There is a conspicuous new awareness that people with dementia have different levels of insight and that, whatever the level, they are able to respond to their environments, both physical and social. The person with dementia is moving to the centre of the stage. This is not always easy for the carer to deal with. Some carers' groups are very uncomfortable with what they see as the hijacking of their organisations by professionals who are as keen to stress the needs of the person with dementia as the needs of carers. Some carers have only been able to cope by believing that their relative is brain dead and beyond responding in any positive way. Many carers have overprotected their relative and feel very uncomfortable with the suggestion that there may be unused cognitive potential and thereby improvement in functioning. This is not unique to relatives. Many, many staff cope by doing everything for the person with dementia or by overuse of medication.

What is being emphasised increasingly is the possibility of empathy with the person with dementia and the possibility of affecting their behaviour for the better by changing the buildings they live in or the way people interact with them. In other words we are beginning to understand that there may be a residual rationality with which we can work. We have always known, even if we did not recognise it, that people with dementia do have some, though usually very minimal, learning skills. They are, for example, able to learn which staff they like and even the way round a ward or day centre.

Some examples will clarify the point. The best examples relate to behaviour, which is the main issue in the care of a person with dementia. In a sense the diagnosis of dementia in itself means relatively little, it is the resultant behaviour which needs attention. We used to assume that behaviour was the result of the deterioration of the brain. We are increasingly aware that it is the result of the inter-relationship of the disease and the social and buildings environment. We now know, for example, that buildings can be made more understandable for people with dementia and that they are then more independent (Coles *et al.* 1992). We used to think of wandering as a symptom of dementia which had to be allowed for. We now know that there are several types of wandering and that some of them are the result of genuinely wanting to go somewhere, others a result of boredom or frustration, and a few defy explanation. We know that if we can make building design sufficiently orientating and engaging we can reduce anxiety and allow opportunities for exercise. We also know that if we provide sufficient activities we can reduce boredom and frustration. Indeed, some recent authors (Fleming 1991, Peppard 1991) maintain that in their units wandering ceases because of the design and regime. Peppard (1991) calls wandering a myth.

Psychologists have led the way with behaviour management and there are plenty of excellent books such as the Winslow Press series (Stokes 1988). However it has taken a while for the implications to hit service providers: that people with dementia can respond to therapeutic input. The CADE units in New South Wales (Fleming 1991) are specialist units which cater for people with severe behaviour problems. They have found that they can dramatically reduce these problems and can, in addition, resurrect old skills by using a specially designed, domestic style and highly interactive regime. The activities are familiar domestic activities because there are no domestic staff and each patient has a carefully formulated care plan. Patients actually improve in spite of having dementia, although they ultimately deteriorate physically and mentally as the disease proceeds toward death.

The implications of this new approach to people with dementia are the same for social workers as they are for any other paid or unpaid carer: that we have to involve people with dementia and that we have to direct therapeutic work towards them. The National Consumer Council produced a very influential report in the 1980s showing how people with dementia could be consumers with a view on their services.

This trend towards seeing the behaviour normally ascribed to the dementia disease process as, instead, a way of coping with the disease and the environment will be helped by the increasing numbers of books where people with dementia actually explain why they behave as they do. These are people in the early stages but they give a fascinating glimpse into the demented mind. Bob Davis (1989) explains that he needs to walk as a way of orientating himself. He claims that knowing who he is and where he is is greatly assisted by having his feet on the floor and walking about. He says he cannot stand too much stimulation; it makes him very tired and he takes days to recover. He says he cannot tell the difference between dreams and reality, which makes him fearful and anxious. Several people with dementia in Naughtin and Laidler's book (1991) explain their high levels of anxiety and fear, and in some cases how they coped with them.

It is obviously impossible to empathise with a person with dementia except for odd flashes. We have, for example, all walked into rooms and wondered why we are there. We have all woken up wondering where we are. We have all panicked when we have forgotten something, most usually a name. We have all become irrationally angry and upset when we have been lost. We are beginning to see the extent to which fear and anxiety play a part in the behaviour of people with dementia and how quickly their confidence and self esteem is demolished. Kitwood (1990) takes this further. He asserts that it is the way that the person with dementia is treated which so undermines their competence.

This new empathy and awareness of the origins of the behaviour of people with dementia is going to increase. In many ways it is very helpful in making our services more sensitive. It also gives us all more responsibility and thereby more stress. It makes huge demands on us to interact in an empathetic manner, which is difficult and demanding.

COMMUNICATION

The best work with people with dementia takes account of the person they were before and the person they now are, with a failing memory, diminished ability to think rationally and so on. It is a disease that makes communication very difficult. It is extremely hard to know how much of the memory or other abilities have been wiped out. They often cannot tell you whether they like one pillow or two, or whether they like Chopin, Mahler or Big Band. They often cannot tell you whether they can still do something. Communication is frequently indirect, with a high feeling content. People with dementia have feelings like any of us, and they are often very intense. They can, for example, be clearly unhappy but be unable to tell you that it is because someone has sugared their tea and they do not take sugar, or someone is playing Scottish country dance music and they hate it. (Using music in two examples is deliberate because the enjoyment of music outlasts most other functions of the brain.) We have a chapter on reminiscence that addresses the need for this degree of knowledge in order to understand and properly plan care in a longstay setting.

The person doing the caring has to take 95 per cent of the responsibility for any interaction. They usually have to initiate activity because people with dementia tend to be apathetic. They have to translate communications constantly, whether they be verbal or not. It has been suggested that having dementia is like being in a world where everybody is speaking a different language. From the paid or unpaid carers' point of view it is as if the person with dementia were speaking a different language. They may communicate allegorically. In other words they tell a story which illustrates what they are trying to say. Thus they may talk about wanting to go home which may be a way of saying they do not understand why they are where they are. They may weep for a lost friend as a way of saying they feel bereft. The key must be knowing the individual. Many professionals are caring for shadows. They have no idea about the family, the jobs, the interests, the degree of religious conviction, the musical tastes and so on. Without this knowledge the translation job is near impossible because you have no clues at all. It is like talking to a naked eskimo with no idea where she comes from. Fortunately, records are improving all the time, with good forms that list biographical detail and preferences. Life story books are increasingly talked about. (This is a technique lifted from child care with children who have little sense of self – a straight parallel.)

Having said that we are getting more expert at communication, it has to be repeated that this is a very demanding kind of work, especially if it is done well. On top of the constant need to be taking the initiative, being creative and responding to feelings, is the sadness that underlies a lot of this work. People with dementia are dying. The more love and attention you invest in giving them the best quality of life, the more you grieve when they die.

STAFF SURVIVAL

Staff need a lot of reassurance and recognition that they are doing a very difficult and skilled job. They need to know if they are doing it well. They need good supervision in order to reflect on their work and to be as purposeful and creative as possible. Problem solving is often best done in twos or in a group and there are lots of problems to work on. Staff need time to cry and, perhaps surprisingly, to laugh because the mis-communications and misunderstandings can be hilarious, but it would be unkind to laugh with the person with dementia. Staff need to be able not to work with people with dementia if they are feeling low.

We need to begin to address the need for sabbaticals or study leave in order to recharge batteries. We may need to accept that it is not realistic to work in this field for more than three years full-time without a substantial break. The time would be longer, obviously, for field staff who are not in full-time contact with the clients, but burnout will happen and needs to be recognised. Constant training and retraining are a way to reduce burnout because they provide new ideas, validation of existing skills and time out. All this applies to unpaid carers too although the struggle to know a stranger is less, the grief can be much greater. Not every relationship has been straightforward and positive, relatives often carry a great deal of ambivalence and unfinished business into the caring role.

DILEMMAS

This field is full of dilemmas and the more knowledgeable we become, the more dilemmas we face. It was, for instance, much easier in the past to assume that the person with dementia had lost the capacity to feel anything. We were able to tolerate the appalling standards in some settings without too much anxiety. We were also much more relaxed about giving priority to the needs of relatives. This is no longer possible. We are now fully aware of the conflict of interests that, more often than not, arise. We are going to have to develop techniques, such as negotiating, in order to work this out and get the 'best possible' deal for both parties. This is covered in *Working with Dementia* (Marshall 1989). What is different is that we now have the full weight of the community care legislation and its local arrangements which are based on the assumption that there is a confluence of interests.

Another dilemma which does not go away is that of integration versus segregation. There are no easy answers, more a list of pros and cons. The pros for integration are the maintenance of the person with dementia in a normal setting and the chance for people who are fearful of their own future seeing the courteous and purposeful care they can expect if they get dementia. The cons are the hostility that alert residents can feel to people with dementia, especially if they do not know and care about them. Those with dementia can also be seen to be making unreasonable demands on staff and as disruptive and disturbing. The people with dementia can become isolated and scapegoated. It is the behaviour, rather than the person, that is the problem. Cheerful, likeable and attractive people with dementia can fit well into day care and longstay care with alert people and be much appreciated. However, people who rummage in other people's drawers, or become sexually disinhibited are a different matter.

The pros for segregation, whether of alert people or of those with dementia, are that there is a specialised environment where expectations are less high (and anxieties thereby diminished) and a regime geared to meeting specific needs. The cons are that units for people with dementia can quickly go down hill. They can be stigmatised. Staff can be exhausted. Standards can drop. Ideally, we need both options. On the whole, we need every longstay and day care setting to have sub units for people with challenging behaviour. A sub unit enables clients to share activities when appropriate, and staff to have time off the unit.

One of the most difficult issues is whether or not to move people as their needs change. The relocation research which has traditionally been read as indicating that moves were in themselves bad for frail older people is now coming up with examples (Hardwood and Ebrahim 1992) where there were no ill effects as long as the move was accompanied by familiar staff and was to improved conditions. Most carers would like their relatives to remain in one place until they die: usually at home but, if not, then in one longstay setting. But can any one setting cope with the changing needs as the disease progresses? Can any one setting provide the stimulation needed in the middle stages, the regime that is needed for challenging behaviour and the hospice type care that is needed at the end? This has not been resolved but may become clearer with the increasing use of multi-factor assessments, which give a full picture of the needs of the person with dementia at any point. As well as providing a tool for allocation to the setting, these assessment measures also enable progress to be monitored to see that the setting is being as effective as possible.

Related to this is the dilemma of whether to move staff. I have shared my views about staff burnout but did not mention the fact that this can have a negative affect on the person with dementia who, above all else, needs staff who know and care for her and provide that familiarity that is so crucially important to people with very impaired learning skills. Yet staff, after an optimum period, become less and less effective. Perhaps we should only have part time staff but this means the person with dementia has to learn more faces. There is no answer but, as with conflict of interest with carers, this has to be confronted and the 'best possible' outcome achieved.

CONCLUSIONS

Dementia is a terrible disease which causes great distress to families and friends. Our state of knowledge and our skills are, however, developing rapidly to meet the challenge. Social workers have plenty to offer in making the pathway through the disease, for the person and for the carers, as easy as it can be. It is important to be optimistic. It is even more important to remember that the person with dementia is first a person and second a person with a disease of the brain.

REFERENCES

Coles, R., Duncan, I., Kelly, M., Marshall, M. and Whiteman, A. (1992) *Signposts not Barriers*. Stirling: Dementia Services Development Centre.

Davis, R. (1989) *My Journey Through Alzheimer's Disease*. Illinois: Tyndale House Publishers.

Feil, N. (1992) *Validation The Feil Method, How to Help Disorientated Old-Old*. Ohio: Edward Feil Productions.

Fleming, R. (1991) *Issues of Assessment and Design in Longstay Care*. Stirling: Dementia Services Development Centre.

Hardwood, R.H. and Ebrahim, B. (1992) Is Relocation Harmful to Institutionalised Elderly People? *Age and Ageing* 21, 61–66.

Jorm, A.F. and Korten, A.E. (1986) A Method for Calculating Projected Increases in the Number of Dementia Sufferers. *Australian and New Zealand Journal of Psychiatry* 22, 183–189.

Kitwood, T. (1990) The Dialectics of Dementia with Particular Reference to Alzheimer's Disease. *Ageing and Society* 18, 177–196.

Mace, N.L., Rabins, P.V., Castleton, B.A., Cloke, C. and McEwen, E. (1985) *The Thirty Six Hour Day*. Age Concern England.

Marshall, M. (ed) (1989) *Working With Dementia*. Birmingham: Venture Press.

National Health Service, Health Advisory Service (1982) *The Rising Tide: Developing Services for Mental Illness in Old Age*. Sutton: Health Advisory Service.

Naughtin, G. and Laidler, T. (1991) *When I Grow Too Old to Dream*. Australia: Collins Dove.

Peppard, N.R. (1991) *Special Needs Dementia Units: Design, Development and Operations*. New York: Springer Publishing.

Stokes, G. (1988) *Aggression*. Oxon: Winslow Press.

Stokes, G. (1988) *Wandering*. Oxon: Winslow Press.

Stokes, G. (1988) *Screaming and Shouting*. Oxon: Winslow Press.

POINTS FOR DISCUSSION

1. What are the grounds for optimism in working with people with dementia?

2. What was your main area of previous practice and what social work methods did you use? How transferrable is your experience in terms of working with people with dementia and their carers?

3. 'Staff need time to cry and at times to laugh.' Is the same true for carers?

4. What are the pros and cons of segregation in terms of a specialist environment for people with severe dementia?

CHAPTER TWO

Psychotherapeutic Intervention with Individuals and Families where Dementia is Present

Iain Gardner

INTRODUCTION

In many ways there is nothing unique about counselling in situations where one member of the family has a dementia. Most of the skills that the worker utilizes are the same as those that are applicable across the board, whether you are intervening in a case of child maltreatment or assisting a client with the development of improved self esteem. All counsellors will identify a beginning, middle and end phase to their counselling process. They will utilize well developed listening and attending skills and will, more than likely, rely on a conceptual or theoretical framework on which they base their intervention.

Although the basics of counselling are not unique to the field of dementia, there are a number of significant issues which will have an impact on the way in which the counselling is conducted when there is a client with dementia.

The provision of counselling to individuals or families where dementia is present relies on the worker having a thorough working knowledge of dementia and the implications that this will have for all those involved. It is disadvantageous to separate out the varying roles that a worker may take with a family where dementia has been diagnosed. That is, the therapeutic role should not be undertaken by a different person from that who provides the practical education, support and advocacy roles. This, however, assumes that the worker has the generic skills to successfully undertake all of these roles to the benefit of the client. Where this is not possible it is in the best interests of the client for the worker to make a referral to the most appropriate other worker best able to meet the client's needs. By centralizing the roles into one worker the client is prevented from having yet another person involved, with possibly another organization to relate to. This centralization also assists the worker in optimizing their therapeutic intervention. This will be discussed further.

Workers who counsel in the field of dementia should not judge themselves too harshly, since they are pioneers in a new field. Dementia has come more to the fore in the last ten years, with a relatively small body of knowledge available for those who are interested. The arena of counselling in the field displays a gross lack of literature available for use by practitioners searching for guidance. Much of what workers counselling in this field experience can be viewed as a parallel process to that which people caring for a person with dementia experience. That is, much of what they do is based on trial and error. They are presented with a problem for which there is no known remedy within their existing bag of tricks and new and often creative ideas must be explored. Carers are often very inventive in the ways in which they deal with the everyday problems that dementia presents. Counsellors equally need to be inventive in their application of techniques to assist clients to resolve some of their emotional problems as they arise.

The possibilities available to workers are endless. It is important that each individual worker find a style that fits with their personality and way of operating. There is no point in a worker using the techniques associated with psychodrama if this is going to cause them great discomfort. It has been my experience that, historically, little in the way of counselling has been done with older adults. When it has been carried out it has, more than likely, been of a very traditional and conservative style designed to resolve a practical problem. It is not often considered that older adults experience the same psychological problems as the rest of the population as well as having the additional burden of the ageing process and, of more relevance here, of dementia.

It has been my experience that older adults respond well, like the rest of the population, to a range of therapeutic modalities which should be tailored to meet their individual needs. Provided that workers acknowledge their professional ethics, work within the basic counselling frameworks and have access to quality supervision, they should feel free to experiment with the application of a range of therapeutic techniques when dealing with issues of dementia.

THE THERAPY PROCESS

The therapy process, no matter what modality is used, is similar to most other processes. It is circular and cyclic in nature. The process can be summarized in the following diagrammatic manner:

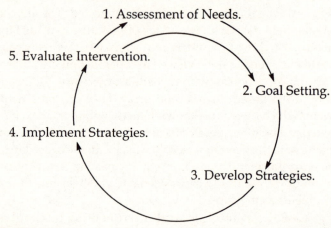

1. Assessment of Needs.

5. Evaluate Intervention.

2. Goal Setting.

4. Implement Strategies.

3. Develop Strategies.

ASSESSMENT

The assessment stage is crucial in determining the success or otherwise of the intervention with a family where dementia is present. Often very little time is devoted to the assessment phase and workers launch straight into the therapeutic intervention. This is very easy to do as the client, as an individual or as a family, will be likely to present with a plethora of issues.

Nonetheless, the reins of enthusiasm must be drawn in and time set aside for the development of a good working diagnosis of the issues. My experience indicates that the assessment process alone is often very therapeutic for the client. Often this is the first time that the client (individual or family) has actually worked through the illness and its impact on them in a systematic way. When this is done within the safety of a well developed client/worker relationship, it has the potential to shape the way in which the client will deal with the rest of their encounters with you as a therapist. This will become more evident when we discuss the actual needs of clients throughout the course of the illness process.

Regardless of whether the presenting problem is a complex, psychodynamic, family problem or it is the preparation for residential care, it is essential that the worker has a working knowledge of the psychosocial situation of the client. When assessing individuals, couples, families or groups where dementia is present it is important to get a total picture of the functioning, both present and past. It is essential, however, to investigate the following:

- medical assessment of person with dementia
- family and social networks
- life cycle stage of all concerned
- social and economic situation
- previous ways of dealing with a crisis
- perceptions of the problem
- what has brought them to seek help at this time
- current functioning of all concerned

It is possible to gather much of this information in a very relaxed and informal way. If, as is usually the case, the initial meeting is post diagnosis of the illness, then it is likely that they will already have been through a barrage of formal tests, questions and interviews. In order for them to see the worker as a real human being it is important that a non-clinical approach is taken which will set you apart from the many medical professionals that have already dealt with them. This is often much easier to do within the client's own home, where you are not restricted by the confines of an office. When a client talks about the difficulty that they are experiencing in the bath it is beneficial for you to get them to show you exactly what they mean in the bathroom.

This gives you not only a solid and concrete understanding of the problem as it is encountered, but also consolidates the relationship by allowing the client to share a real and solid part of themselves with you. Interviewing within the client's own home also allows for a greater deal of flexibility in dealing with people who have dementia and who may have behavioural problems. In summary, workers should try, wherever possible to interview clients within their own homes. This is especially important in the early stages when the assessment is being conducted and a trusting relationship developed.

At this stage the worker has gathered a lot of information which aims to give them a better understanding of the client's potential and limitations. This is only the first part of the assessment process. The second stage of the process is that which separates the information gatherer from the professional practitioner. That is the development of a diagnostic or an assessment statement.

The assessment statement develops from the information gathered and pulls together the psychosocial information with the current problems as assessed and agreed upon by both client and worker. This statement usually forms part of the psychosocial report and lends itself to the development of specific change goals. This is the stage where concrete goals are formed and solid roots set for the intervention.

In spending a considerable amount of time with one family who presented for counselling because of conflict between the siblings in regard to the care of their mother who had dementia, the assessment process revealed that no time had been spent on providing the family with the basic information about the illness. A misunderstanding about the genetic inheritance of the disease had resulted in such a high stress level in both sisters that they were in conflict with each other about nothing of significance. Gaining a thorough understanding of where they were all coming from, and where they were all at, enabled me to meet their real needs by providing them with some basic education rather than launching into counselling to explore their sibling rivalry. This does not, however, mean that there was not in fact a problem between the sisters but rather that it had manifested itself due to another problem. In this case no further problem between them occurred in the course of their care for their mother; however, it very easily could have. Assessment is vital in establishing the priorities which will be worked with. Given that dementia often results in multiple problems for a family it is important that the worker has a place to start.

GOAL SETTING

The establishment of goals flows on very easily from a solid assessment which contains a diagnostic statement. If this first stage has been done correctly then there will already be clear targets for change. By asking the simple question 'what do we want to achieve from undertaking counselling?' we are in fact setting our targets.

Many counsellors have one set of targets that are identified by their clients and another set for themselves which are not always articulated. For example, in the previous case, one worker may have set the objective to educate the family about the illness and may have run with an agenda to look later at the sibling problem. I have a preference to keep all of my objectives up front and gain acceptance from the client. In this case I clearly articulated that I felt that the problem between the sisters was secondary to the lack of education and that we should explore that first. If a problem still existed between them, then we could do some more exploration around the issue. (My way of operating is more in line with the humanistic style of counselling where less reliance is placed on the unconscious work of the client.)

Once worker and client have agreed on the priority of the problems that are going to be worked on, the changed objectives are set. The goals should be directly related to the identified problems and should aim to reduce the difficulty and the associated stress of the problem. This may sound very straightforward; however, it never ceases to amaze me the number of times that I find myself asking workers in supervision 'Why are you doing that?'. Often they cannot answer the question. Again, because of the abundance of problems that could be apparent, or the ones that often surface anew when undergoing counselling, it is important to plan. When counselling people with dementia and their families, failing to plan is planning to fail!

These goals, which are always aimed at improving functioning, should be concrete and specific. Both the client and the worker must understand what is meant by the objective. If they are concrete and specific then they should easily lend themselves to evaluation. Examples of non-specific objectives include the following common requests; I want to be happy; I want to come to terms with the disease; I want to get over her death. These objectives do not lend themselves to strategy development and it is not easy to evaluate the client's success in achieving them. Often it is easy to let the client get away with being this vague rather than helping them to clearly identify what, specifically, they want. As mentioned previously, this process is often in itself therapeutic and assists the client to be responsible in identifying their needs.

The clients should be lead with comments such as: What would need to change to make you happier? What does 'come to terms with the disease' mean for you? What is it about your mother's death that causes you the greatest concern? The client is assisted and prompted to be clear and specific about the problem and what has to be different for them to feel better.

Examples of clear and specific cases which could result after further prompting could include: 'I want to be able to sleep better at nights, I want to be able to understand what is going to happen to me as the disease progresses, I want to deal with the guilt that I experience because I put Mum in a nursing home'. These are far more concrete but could still be further refined down to specific points. Perhaps there will be many specific objectives which grow from the original global one. When the objectives become this concrete and specific they flow into the development of strategies.

STRATEGY DEVELOPMENT

When clients have been assisted in identifying their own objectives down to the specifics, they are often able to identify the strategies that are required. This is another reason why it is important for the worker to spend time assessing the needs and developing strategies. The strategies are the means to the end. It is how we assist the client to move from point A to B. Like the objectives, the strategies should be concrete and specific. These are actions which need to be tied to time lines. The strategies are the actions that will be undertaken to result in the improved functioning of the client.

The strategies will include: who will be involved in the process to bring about the change; who or what will need to change or be influenced in order to meet the objectives, and who is going to benefit from the change. It is important when dealing with dementia to be very clear about who the actual client is. Sometimes these roles get blurred and the objectives of different members within the system are not congruent with each other.

IMPLEMENTATION OF STRATEGIES

There is little point in undertaking all of this assessment and planning and leaving it at that. That is, of course, unless, as is sometimes the case, this has been enough to bring about change. More often than not, however, the worker and client do not get off that lightly and well developed strategies need to be auctioned.

It is here that the worker puts into place the therapeutic skills to successfully achieve the set objectives. The tools and roles that the worker utilizes are many and varied and will be discussed in more detail later.

EVALUATION

The purpose of this stage of the process is to measure how successful the strategies have been in meeting the objectives. In the field of counselling, evaluation has only just started to gain its rightful place. For too long it has been placed in the 'too hard' basket, or more likely into the 'too frightening' basket.

In counselling, the evaluation process should not be left to the last minute, but rather should continue throughout the intervention. This is particularly important where dementia is involved, as the changes associated with the disease process require that the worker be responsive to the changing needs of the client.

The evaluation process is a reassessment of the situation and flows into the adjustment of the goals and strategies to be used in the future. It is a time to see what has worked to the benefit of the client and what did not work so well. As previously mentioned, much of the work with families where dementia is present is new and the techniques are substantially untested in the field. As such, the evaluation process is imperative to the development of skills.

Although very little attention has been given to the evaluation of psychotherapy, more literature is becoming available and techniques can be developed to assess success. It is more difficult to assess the longer term benefits to clients who have been helped through the dementia process but if the goals which are set are concrete and measurable then the evaluation need only measure against these.

Workers should build the evaluation process into their contracts with clients. That is, clients should be informed that evaluation will take place within a nominated session and should be assisted to set evaluation indications. The final session in the contracted group of sessions should be devoted to re-evaluating the situation, setting new goals, strategies and time lines. This process insures that both worker and client stay on track and remain responsive to the current need.

Post counselling sessions: there are a number of ways that a worker can assess the effectiveness of the intervention. Given the long term nature of dementia it is possible for workers to contract with clients for follow up at a nominated point in the future. This serves the dual purpose of providing a mechanism for longterm evaluation and provides the client with a safety net in case of future issues requiring assistance. For those clients who do not have a future contract with the worker it is possible to follow up with a questionnaire designed to gain feedback of the client's perspective on the impact of the intervention.

DEMENTIA

As we are aware, the behaviour of a person with dementia is unpredictable. The disease itself, however, is somewhat more predictable. Although no two people display exactly the same changes due to the disease, there is a general pattern in the losses associated within the illness. The following table outlines the gradual losses experienced.

At different stages of the illness the needs of the person with dementia and their family and friends will be different. The challenge for the worker is to balance the short and longterm needs of the clients at the same time. For example, it is often difficult to balance the need that a family has in the early stage of the illness for information about what deterioration to expect, with their emotional feelings of loss and grief. Unlike many other forms of counselling where the worker is engaging in one mode or the other, when working with dementia you can be undertaking longterm supportive counselling at the same time as you are dealing with a complex psychodynamic problem in the family and also responding in a crisis framework to a catastrophe.

Although the needs of the client vary according to the stage of the disease, it is essential that workers do not take on a compartmental approach, but rather take a longitudinal view, seeing their involvement as a process. Education about the disease is very much a need associated with the early stage of the illness; however, it must be constantly reinforced and clarified for all concerned along the way. It is essential to remember that if you have dementia or care for someone with dementia then you will be living under a great deal of stress. This necessitates constant reinforcement, affirmation and clarification of understanding about all aspects of the counselling process.

NEEDS AND STAGES

People with dementia can be diagnosed at any stage of the illness. Often the family and the person have noticed changes for a considerable time; it is not, however, until the changes interfere with functioning that assistance is sought. In the past this has resulted in people receiving diagnosis when they have been quite advanced in the disease process. More recently, however, with the great increase in the publicity about

ALZHEIMER'S DISEASE – THE GRADUAL LOSSES

Forgetfulness

Word Finding Problems

Mild confusion

Anxiety

Mild Personality
Changes

Depression

Inability to Learn
New Things

Paranoid Thoughts

Increasing Memory
Problems

Obsessional Behaviours

Repetitive
Questioning

Problems with Making Decisions

Disorientation in
Time, Place
and Person

Reservation

Decreasing
Communication

Loss of Forward Planning

Problems with Self Care

Decreased Independence in
Activities of Daily Living

Poor Problem Solving

Agitation, Restlessness
and Wandering

Incontinence Problems

Behavioural Problems

Sleep Disturbances

Falls

Language Loss and
Communication Problems

Loss of Identity

Extreme Disorientation

Extreme Confusion

Confined to bed

Double Incontinence

No Communication

No Mobility

Major Loss of All Functioning

Death

dementia, people are more aware of the disease and its early indicators. This has resulted in very early detection of the disease. The stage at which diagnosis is made will, to a certain extent, determine the counselling needs at that time.

PRE-DIAGNOSIS

With the increased information and publicity available about dementia a 'dementia paranoia' has developed. Conversations at parties joke about having dementia. Information services take many calls from people wanting diagnostic information because they think they may have the disease. Given that the early symptoms of dementia are similar to the symptoms of stress and depression, it is essential that workers are able to assess the psychosocial situation of the person to eliminate these as the cause of the symptoms. One must be mindful, however, that experiencing the early symptoms of dementia can in itself result in stress and depression. This is where a good working knowledge of the illness is required in order to pick up indicators for referral for a medical assessment.

At this stage clients often require basic information about the illness and the assessment and support services available. If a medical assessment is indicated it is often necessary to guide the client through the process and to support them on an emotional level. Often the client will want to know about the types of tests that will be carried out, so it is beneficial for the worker to be well informed about the assessment process utilized.

Often at this stage the client is a family member who is concerned about someone in the family displaying symptoms. Here the worker is often required, in addition to working through the issues for the client, to assist them in developing strategies to get their family member assessed. This requires incredible creativity and sensitivity as this is usually the first of many changes in the established roles within the family that a person will have to make as they become the carer of someone with dementia. The client will need to be assisted in the transition from the role of child or spouse to that of carer. This often involves significant changes in the existing relationships and sometimes involves breaking family rules. Active and reflective listening skills are required as the worker displays empathy, acknowledges feelings and guides the client to their own solutions.

Also at this stage clients may need to be taught how to work the system. They need to know what services are available and how they can access them. Frequently clients will need to be taught how to be assertive when dealing with the health and welfare system.

For those clients who present with symptoms of some other illness or psychological disorder, it will be necessary for them to be referred to the most appropriate agency. This requires a good knowledge of the available community resources. The worker must have a knowledge of normal and abnormal behaviours and the diagnostic skills to separate these from the dementia process.

EARLY STAGE

The most frequent need that clients present with in following diagnosis is for information about the illness. They may have been given the basic information about the illness at this time, but it is unlikely that they will have taken much in as their cognitive functioning will have been impaired by the stress of the diagnosis. By systematically working through with the client what they do and do not know, the worker is establishing a relationship and is gathering valuable information for the assessment. It is important at this stage that the worker reflects and acknowledges the emotional reactions and not only the content of the discussion. The client will have a strong need to test their reactions for sanity and wherever possible these should be normalised and affirmed.

By providing clients with a good working knowledge of the disease process at this early stage and preparing them with a general framework about what to expect, it is possible to minimize the impact that the unexpected changes would have. For example, the period when a person becomes incontinent is often seen as a crisis point in the process. If clients are aware that this is likely to occur at some stage and have a basic knowledge of the services which are available to assist them, then the crisis will be minimised.

In the early stages of the illness people with dementia and their carers require assistance with planning on a practical level. They need help with working the system, in financial and legal matters whilst the person with dementia is still competent and they may need to explore practical care issues. At this stage the worker's knowledge of practical care hints is most valuable. This is particularly important if changes need to take place to ensure smoother care in the future. As the disease progresses the ability of the person with dementia to learn new things decreases dramatically. As such, any new learning should be planned for in the very early stage. For example, many carers find it beneficial to use a whiteboard system to write messages and cues for the day. Unless this has been a normal daily practice the person with dementia will have to learn this as new. This will be impossible later in the illness.

As previously mentioned, the early stages of the disease is when the first role changes begin to take place. There are the practical issues of the husband who has never cooked before, the wife who has never managed the finances or the daughter who has to prompt her father to take a bath. The actual practicalities of these issues are often easily learnt and solved; however, the emotional responses and the necessary mind shift required are more daunting.

My experience indicates that by acknowledging these changes with clients, the worker is validating their emotions and providing them with an opportunity to vent their feelings in a setting where they will not be judged. There are no easy answers to these issues as we are attempting to get clients to operate systems which change the very systems and sub-systems of families that much of our therapy is designed to preserve. As such we can only allow clients to ventilate their emotions and to assist them in clarifying the issues as they relate to them.

The issue of loss and grief is probably the single most significant issue when dealing with people with dementia and their carers. This issue will be dealt with as a separate item later in the chapter, but it must be stressed that the grief reaction will begin as soon as, if not before the diagnosis of the disease is made.

The diagnosis of dementia generates a stress reaction within families. This can be the trigger for unleashing any unfinished business that exists. As such a worker in this field cannot expect their work to be confined to the issues of dementia. In one case where I was working with a family where the mother had dementia, it became very obvious in the very early stages of the assessment that something else was going on between two of the daughters. It turned out they had both been carrying around some unfinished business for thirty years about one of the daughters seducing and subsequently marrying the other's boy friend. The crisis of having to come together to plan for their mother's care triggered this reaction.

The principle of immediacy is required in a situation such as this. That is, when something comes up in the counselling situation that prevents the achievement of set goals, then that problem must be dealt with first. In this case I could have suggested that we were not here to discuss the issue of thirty years ago and that we should get on with the problem at hand. Instead, what I did was to look at that issue from the past as it was affecting the current situation. By reliving the past situation and getting them to say all of the things that they had wanted to say but had never got round to, they resolved a longterm dispute which consolidated their relationship and also enabled them to work harmoniously on the plans for the provision of care for their mother. This case highlights only one of the many issues that can surface when a family is confronted with dementia. What this even more clearly highlights is the need for the worker to deal with whatever comes up for the client.

Early intervention with people with dementia and their carers which provides information, education, emotional support, practical advice and counselling as required will prevent the client from going from crisis to crisis. What happens early in the disease process will shape what will happen later.

MIDDLE STAGE

By the time a person reaches the middle stage of the dementia process they will be displaying marked changes in their personality and ability to care for themselves. Behavioural problems will usually develop and, later in the stage, incontinence. This stage can be classified as the dependency stage. The person with dementia is dependent on somebody else for their physical care and for their thinking and problem solving.

The marked change in personality and behaviour most often causes the greatest difficulty for carers at this stage. Carers grapple with the change in the person from the person that they once knew. This problem is exacerbated by the overlay of the physical dependence and often the tiredness of the primary carer due to lack of sleep.

It is usually at this stage that a decision is required in regard to where the person with dementia will be cared for. Will they be managed at home or will institutional care be required? Historically, in Australia at least, the casework practice for residential care (or placement work, as it is often referred) has been regarded as low status and purely practical. Until recently, the social workers undertaking this work have been new graduates with little or no counselling experience. The complex psychodynamics of such work has often not been identified, much less dealt with.

More recently, the importance of a counselling framework for residential work has been acknowledged. This is still quite inadequate considering the massive life decisions being made under stress. Whilst working at the Alzheimer's Society of Victoria I noted that a significant number of referrals were made for counselling for people who had placed their relative with dementia into care approximately 18 months or two years before. It was at this time that problems re-presented. I refer to this as 'post placement trauma'.

The move into residential care is one of the most significant stages in the life cycle for both the person moving and the carers. The issues of guilt and grief are usually paramount and if not properly addressed will result in dysfunction later in life. A significant amount of time should be devoted to preparing families for the move and to give them the opportunity to explore both their positive and negative feelings. They will require follow up as placement is not the end of the road, but rather the beginning of a new set of issues and concerns.

At this stage of the illness it is obvious that clients will be experiencing large amounts of stress. As such the role of the worker is to assist them in developing strategies to deal with this.

END STAGE

By now the person with dementia will be totally dependent and will little resemble the person that they used to be. The end result is death. It is at this stage that many workers discharge their clients and send them back into the world. It is important to remember that clients are likely to have been caring for the person for a number of years and it is probable that dementia has become a major part of their life. The task of the worker at this stage is to assist the client, not only to deal with their grief, but also to get their life back to normal and to reintegrate into society.

Many carers state that they have forgotten how to speak to 'normal' people. They have often become socially isolated and detached from mainstream society. The major issues to be confronted include developing staff confidence and self esteem, reestablishing social networks and dealing with the loss and grief.

SOME OF THE MAJOR ISSUES

Guilt

Carers constantly talk about feeling guilty about a range of issues. 'I feel guilty because: I should have cared for him at home; I am spending her money; I went out last night and left her alone; I wish he were dead', and so on.

Guilt, unfortunately, is not a very concrete or tangible emotion. I ask clients the questions; 'When you feel guilty, how do you feel? Where do you feel it: in your body?' I do not believe that guilt exists as a gut emotion but rather that it is a syndrome of other emotions. Most often when clients talk about guilt they are actually feeling angry or sad. These feelings are not as socially acceptable and guilt is much safer. By helping clients to identify and articulate what they are feeling heightens their personal awareness and becomes the basis for any change that may be required. It is difficult to initiate change outside of true awareness.

In association with guilt is the client who constantly talks of shoulds. 'I should do this; I should have done that, or I should not feel this'. Shoulds are indicators of introjections. These are messages, values, behaviours or the like that we take in whole from our environment (usually from our parents) that do not necessarily fit with what we really want to do, think or feel. Clients can be assisted in working out where their shoulds come from and then assessing whether they in fact do fit with their own values. If the client can replace the 'should' with 'want to', there is no problem. It is my experience that often just by raising the use of 'should' to the client's awareness is sufficient to start them on the questioning of their motivation for saying and doing particular things.

Loss

The word dementia is almost interchangeable with the word loss. The disease process is about a gradual loss in functioning and the deterioration of a person's personality. The loss of your very being must be the most significant loss that anyone can suffer. For the carer, as well as the person with dementia there are many losses. The worker can assist the client in identifying and articulating these losses. It is important to investigate what other losses the client has had in their life and how they dealt with them. A loss now can trigger the feelings associated with previous losses and how previous losses were dealt with will determine the client's preferred way of dealing with this loss.

Often, because of dementia, the carer cannot talk through their loss with their loved one. This can result in much unfinished business. In this instance it is beneficial to use the empty chair technique where the worker assists the client to pretend that the other person is sitting in an empty chair opposite them. They should be encouraged to enter into dialogue with each other to enact the unfinished situation. This technique is beneficial in situations where the client does not have the ability to talk to another person or wishes to practice their interaction first.

Much has been written about loss and grief counselling and workers in the field of dementia will have a need to familiarise themselves with the theory and practice.

Self-determination

Most counsellors, especially social workers, are preached to about client self-determination and how to maintain it for our clients. Dementia raises the question: at what stage in the process of the illness do we acknowledge that a person with dementia is not competent to self determine their own life? This generates both ethical and legal questions for workers. Do we allow the woman with dementia who leaves the gas on, has falls, smokes in bed and is incontinent of urine and faeces to remain at home alone because she wants to?

There is no simple answer to this question for workers. It becomes an issue of being familiar with your own professional ethics and the stance of your employing agency on the issue. It is important to remember, however, that people with dementia will have a span of skills which will vary from task to task. As such, a person with dementia may not be capable of self-determining in regard to where they should live but may be able to self-determine about what they would like to wear. Workers should consider carefully their stance in regard to self-determination as they are dealing with vulnerable people without a strong legal or ethical framework for support.

Sex

People over the age of fifty do have sex! There are taboos about talking about it but it happens; thank goodness. The issues of sex in older life have until recently gone unaddressed by workers in the field. Fortunately, workers in the geriatric speciality are now beginning to address the sexual issues of their clients. In the area of dementia, sex manifests itself in a variety of ways. Classically, people think of the man with dementia who becomes sexually disinhibited. This does happen sometimes, but there are many other sexual issues that the worker will be more likely to confront. I remember raising the issue of sex with one woman carer who was grateful at being given the opportunity to discuss it. I expected the sort of problem that I outlined above, but instead she was concerned about her husband's impotence and the resulting frustration for both of them. Lesson number one is that the worker should just sit back and listen to the client.

The task of the worker is to include sexual functioning as a standard part of the psychosocial assessment. It has been my experience that clients respond to the opportunity to discuss sexual issues if they are heard in a safe environment without judgement. It is important to break the conspiracy of silence that exists around sex, particularly in later life.

In dealing with the problems as they present it will be unlikely that workers will have gained much information to help them from their basic training. As such it is important that workers seek out experts in the field to use as consultants to assist them in their intervention or to make referral to if they feel the need.

WHO IS THE CLIENT?

This question often causes workers some difficulty. In the field of dementia it becomes of vital importance as often different members of the system have different needs and expectations. The intervention that a worker chooses may benefit one member of the system and not the other. The issue of identifying the client also has ethical and legal implications.

Client identification may be made easier by organisational limits. For example, in a hospital setting the client is legally determined as the admitted patient. If you are working in a setting where the client is not as easily identified, then it is up to the worker to determine who the client is. Failure to identify your client can result in working at cross purposes with two or more members of the family.

It is important that workers clarify within their agency what the philosophical and legal situation is in regard to the identification of the client. Strong supervision is also beneficial in clarifying who the client is and what implications this will have on the person with dementia. Many would argue that for a client to be a client they must enter into a contract with the worker. In order to enter into a legal contact a person must be mentally competent. As such this would prevent many people with dementia from being viewed as legal clients unless this is conducted via an advocate. The problems associated with this are endless and the worker must remain conscious of the issues at all time.

STRESS

Having dementia or caring for someone who has it generates a great deal of stress. Some of the stressors may be reduced; however, it is more likely that clients will need to explore ways of managing their stress in order to minimise its ill affects.

Often people with dementia and their carers have not identified that they are living with stress so often just acknowledgment of it is beneficial. It is important that clients understand about stress and the effect that it has on their mind and bodies. Clients should be assisted in identifying what it is that stresses them, what their indicators of stress actually are, what are their current adaptive and maladaptive methods of dealing with the stress and new ways of dealing with it.

It is important to remember that clients who are carers will have little time to devote to long stress management techniques so it is important that they are provided with a range of possible exercises that they can adapt to their busy lives. Most stress management books have a number of short mental and physical exercises with which workers can familiarise themselves.

STANDARD LIFE ISSUES

The presence of dementia in a family causes a number of problems in addition to the standard life issues experienced by everyone. These issues require the worker to have a thorough understanding of dementia and its issues, as previously discussed. Nonetheless, it should be remembered that these families also experience all of the standard life issues that other people do.

My experience in counselling families where dementia is present indicates that often many of the presenting problems are quite separate from dementia and have merely been exacerbated or become clarified by the illness process. There is no doubt, however, that the presence of dementia actually complicates the situation and adds yet another dimension that must be managed. As such, the worker in this field must have either generic skills to deal with the plethora of issues that will arise, or high level assessment skills which allow for referral to the most appropriate agency.

SPECIFIC CLIENT GROUPS

People with dementia

As people are obtaining a diagnosis much earlier in the disease process it is becoming imperative that attention is paid to the counselling needs of people with dementia themselves.

It is obviously much easier to work with people in the very early stage of the illness whilst their cognitive ability is not too greatly impaired. It must be remembered that most psychotherapy techniques are designed to be used with healthy individuals. Therefore, when a person has a degree of brain dysfunction, the techniques are less likely to be applicable and will require alteration if they are to meet the client's needs.

In the early stage of the illness the needs of the person with dementia are similar to those of the carer. The grief however, is often more intense as it is their own life and personality that is at stake and they are aware of the burden that they are most likely to become. Whilst the person is still able to process information, the prospect of the future deterioration is very daunting and results not only in anticipatory grief, but also in the reactive depression and a high level of anxiety. This can often exacerbate the symptoms of the disease such as memory loss and confusion.

Apart from the need for information, practical advice and emotional support, the client may require assistance and support in coming to terms with the intensity of their feelings and other's reactions. Here is a time when the worker can use their reflective listening skills to help the client to clarify their thoughts and feelings.

As the person progresses through the disease process, their ability to engage in counselling decreases. This is largely due to decreased memory and problem solving resulting in the inability to learn new things. As counselling is basically about learning new ways to look at things, the process is very difficult for a person with advanced dementia.

Despite this being the case, it should be stressed that although these people cannot actively problem solve, they can feel. It is therefore the task of the worker to respond to the client's feelings. This means being receptive to the nonverbal cues as often the client is not able to communicate their feelings verbally. When workers are receptive they can easily pick up on the anger, sadness and other emotions that the person with dementia experiences. In return, the client may not understand the verbal response of the worker. This is where the neuropsychological assessment can be of assistance in determining the level of functioning. However, it is beneficial for the worker to use non-verbal cues to respond to the client. These must be congruent with what is being said verbally. Remember that even people without dementia when in crisis seldom remember words spoken but remember gestures. The worker needs to smile, use touch and change vocal intonation to communicate effectively.

Wherever possible the person with dementia should be encouraged to be involved in sessions. This not only gives the worker the opportunity to witness the dynamics but also provides a forum for modelling of behaviour and communication with the family in the safety of the counselling session.

The involvement of a person with advanced dementia in a session will require that the worker is creative and patient. There is no doubting that dealing with a person with dementia can sometimes be a trial of your patience so one must be prepared. The involvement should not just be tokenism, but rather must be purposeful and well planned.

A case example illustrates how I learnt this lesson the hard way. I was conducting an initial assessment session with a family in their own home where the elderly mother had quite advanced dementia. They were referred for education and support about caring for their mother at home. The family asked if their mother should be present and I responded that she should. Although I had no clear understanding of why she should be, I did have a philosophical commitment to people with dementia being involved. I had been led to believe by the referring doctor that the woman was in the middle stage of the illness and that her ability to understand and communicate was poor. This was supported by my initial impression on meeting her.

When I got to the stage in the session where it became necessary to provide the family with the basic information about the disease, Daisy, who had until this time been silent, pricked up her ears and looked interested. She said that I was talking too quickly and that she was having trouble keeping up with what I was saying. I very nicely offered her one of my information booklets which explains the disease with all the facts and figures relevant to Victoria and Australia. I told her that everything that I was saying was in the booklet and she could go through it there at her own pace. Basically, I was attempting to distract her to enable me to get on with my real work with the family, when in fact I knew that she would not be able to make any sense of the booklet.

WRONG!! On the first page of the booklet there is a paragraph explaining that Alzheimers is a disease process and that a certain number of people in Australia are affected. Daisy interrupted me and said 'So it's a disease is it?' Shocked, I looked up and replied yes. She then said 'All these people, if they are all as bad as me it will be a sad state of affairs'. From that minute on I have never again assumed anything about people with dementia and I make every effort to involve them in the real process of the session. In this case and many since, I have been able to use the emotional response of the person with dementia as an opener to the emotional responses of other members of the family. In counselling sessions the person with dementia can often be the emotional barometer of the family. They seldom lie and their nonverbals are usually very obvious and accurate.

Women

Dementia is a women's issue. Most people who have dementia are women and most people providing the primary care for someone with dementia are women. I also have a hunch that most people working in the field of dementia care are women also. Workers in the field must work actively to prevent this reinforcement. Sessions must be made available at times when men can attend and the caring role must not be reinforced as a woman's role. At the same time men must be helped to express their emotions about their experiences with dementia. In working in this field it is important that workers are mindful of the social and political implications for women and a feminist approach is useful. As a man in the field I gained a great deal of understanding by discussing the issues with feminist workers. This helps to understand the roles, expectations and demands that many women experience in their roles as carers.

Children

As the incidence of dementia increases, the likelihood of any person not coming in touch with it decreases. Children are included in this and, historically, have received little attention from workers in the field. Children tend to relate well with people with dementia and vice versa. I think that this has something to do with the unconditional love that they can both give and which is generally so difficult to find.

Dementia, however, can be quite scary for children as they struggle to make sense of the unusual behaviours and changing personalities. Children, like adults need to be provided with information appropriate to their level of understanding. They also need the opportunity to voice and work through their thoughts and feelings and to be given some guidance in how best to manage the behaviours.

Young children respond well to creative work using play and art to stimulate discussion. Older children, in particular adolescents, respond well to group intervention. All children should be encouraged to be involved in the counselling process wherever possible. Schools should also be encouraged to educate students about the disease as few will be likely to escape knowing someone with dementia.

SUMMARY AND CONCLUSION

The provision of counselling to people with dementia and their carers requires workers to integrate a large range of skills and roles to produce a generic service which is able to respond to the many, varied and rapidly changing psychosocial needs.

The worker will be called upon to provide education and information, emotional support, practical advice, long and short term psychotherapy and crisis intervention at an individual, couple, family and group level. The issues which present themselves for counselling transcend those directly related to dementia to include practically any psychosocial issue known to counsellors.

Provided that workers plan their intervention based on solid assessments and that they have access to quality supervision, there are endless strategies and techniques which they can apply to meet and set objectives.

Creativity will be required to deal with some of the complicated problems that arise. Workers should not be bound by the traditional constraints of counselling but, at the same time, they should observe the well accepted basic frameworks and principles which underpin the helping process.

Counselling in this field is new and challenging and all workers should be encouraged to document and share their experiences with other practitioners.

REFERENCES

Carter, B. and McGoldrick, M. (eds) (1988) *The Changing Family Life Circle, Second edition*. New York: Gardner Press.

Compton and Galaway (eds) (1978) *Social Work Processes, Revised edition*. USA: Dorsey Press.

Corsini, R.J. (ed) (1989) *Current Psychotherapies, Second edition*. USA: Peacock Publishers.

Gidley, I. and Shears, R. (1987) *Alzheimers*. Australia: Allen and Unwin.

Goding, G. (1992) *The History and Principles of Family Therapy*. Australia: VAFT Publication.

Hoffman, L. (1981) Foundations of Family Therapy. USA: Basic Books

McCallum, P. and Lang, M. (1988) *A Family in Therapy*. Australia: McPhee Gribble Penguin Books.

McGoldrick, M. and Gerson, R. (1985) *Genograms in Family Assessment*. New York: Norton and Company.

POINTS FOR DISCUSSION

1. 'Failing to plan is planning to fail'. Discuss the ways to agree goals that are concrete and specific.

2. Discuss the proposition that an assessment can, in itself, be therapeutic for the client.

3. Consider the problems of engaging in several counselling 'modes' at the same time – for example, in dealing with both long-term and short-term issues.

4. Give examples, and discuss the implications, of likely role changes within the family following the onset of dementia.

5. Is it in your experience true that casework practice in connection for a possible residential placement for people with dementia has had a low status? If so, has the introduction of care in the community procedures (assessment and care management) helped to raise this status?

6. At what stage in the process of dementia do we determine that the person is not competent to self-determine their own life?

7. 'Dementia is a women's issue'. How far is this true and what can be done to include men into the counselling process?

8. Discuss the importance of supervision for staff involved in counselling in the field of dementia. What is the counsellor entitled to expect from supervision?

CHAPTER THREE

The Use of the Past

Faith Gibson

This chapter explores the reasons why the past seems so important and how, for people with dementia, their past may be made to work for them in the present. Three questions will be examined: Why use the past? How can the past be used? What are the practice implications for social workers seeking to use the past?

WHY USE THE PAST?

Our sense of identity, self-esteem and personal confidence is largely rooted in our knowledge of where we have come from and to whom we belong. Crawford *et al.* (1990), Haugh (1987) and Harre (1983) have suggested that memories are the raw material from which our sense of identity and our theories of self are fashioned. Without a consciousness of our past we seem adrift in the present. For almost everyone, a knowledge of the past seems to be crucial to a sense of present well-being. This appears to be true even if we choose, consciously or unconsciously, to set aside or revise this knowledge in order to make our present more acceptable to ourselves and ourselves more interesting to other people (Tarman 1988, Molinari and Reichlin 1984).

Both creative and clinical writing affirms the assertion that knowledge of the past is important to a sense of wellbeing in the present. The strenuous efforts made by survivors of the Nazi Holocaust to seek out even the most tenuous knowledge about their families is well documented. Epstein (1980) and Epstein and Mendelsohn (1978) showed that this process is still continuing long years after the events which led to the loss of family ties.

Other historical and cultural movements leading to the dispossession of people and their resettlement, often in foreign lands have been explored by many writers including Morgan (1991), Haley (1977) and Hewitt (1942). Present security is sought in unravelling the long journey by which their forbears travelled to their family's present geographic and social locations. By knowing the route by which they have come, incomers are able to assert with more confidence that they 'belong'.

Unravelling the past and reaching a present accommodation with it is at the very centre of much therapeutic social work, notwithstanding the contributions of task-centred, time-limited, contractual approaches. In child care, fostering and adoption practice, as McWhenney (1967) and Triseliotis (1973) showed, the past exerts a compelling force. The urge expressed and the actions embarked upon by many adults who were adopted in infancy, or who grew up in care, to find out who their natural parents were is well documented. They have a great need to know and not infrequently to locate the lost parent, even though to do so, they appreciate at a rational level, may possibly lead to further pain and disappointment.

It seems plausible to speculate that if knowledge of our past is important to our sense of wellbeing in the present, it is also important for people with dementia whose hold on the past is becoming more ambiguous, hazy, intermitted and transient.

This speculation is supported by experience with people who in the early stages of dementia are painfully aware, frequently articulate and usually very anxious about their failing memory. Such anxiety seems to be concerned with their decreasing cognitive competence and also with a loss of a sense of connectedness to others which threatens their own identity.

Through careful empathetic listening it is possible, to a limited extent, to put ourselves in these people's shoes. It would be unwise to presume too much about their state of mind but neither should we lightly dismiss what is already known. When professional people diagnose someone as 'confused' or 'demented' it is quite wrong to conclude that the person so labelled is not, to some extent, aware of his or her predicament, and that he or she is untroubled by either the present or the past. Practice experience often suggests exactly the opposite. Observation of many people with dementia suggests that they are profoundly troubled, anxious, restless, frustrated, bewildered and depressed by their inability to 'place' themselves with certainty in the present and to be comfortable with intrusions from the past. The loss of a sense of attachment seems very threatening (Bowlby 1973, Miesen 1992).

For many people with dementia, there are subtle, and not so subtle hints that their past leaks into the present in disturbing and unsettling ways. Most carers see repeated evidence of lost roles, relationships and responsibilities seeping into the present. Much wandering, restlessness and agitation appears to be associated with seeking and searching for the past connections, whether it be as children, wives, spouses, or mothers. Searching for long dead parents or 'parent fixation' is very common. As the dementia progresses many people tend to inhabit increasingly private worlds which exclude others and minimise conversation. So often carers behave in ways which increase this encroaching isolation, reduce communication and accelerate or hasten the retreat into secretive worlds.

Very few people with dementia are totally, continuously or consistently confused. On the contrary, they are partially, intermittently and erratically confused. Instead of being preoccupied with the negative, it is better to use the past to discover what the person still remembers, not what she has forgotten. Assessment needs to focus on what a person can still do, not on what she can no longer do. Exploring the past demonstrates what used to give a person pleasure and satisfaction, and what might possibly still so do. Every negative reaction by the carer to mistake, forgetfulness and lack of comprehension fuels the growing doubts the person has about their cognitive competence and encourages their retreat. Our behaviour encourages their withdrawal.

By its very nature the disease limits knowledge and restricts understanding. It is near impossible for the person with dementia themselves to bear witness. It does, however, seem to resemble a journey from the known, more or less familiar and controllable world which most of us inhabit most of the time, towards a land which is simultaneously familiar and unfamiliar, knowable and unknowable, within control and beyond control.

The challenge to both family and professional carers alike is twofold. How may we become sufficiently acquainted with the person with dementia's old familiar landscape as to be able to recognise its landmarks? How may we show our willingness to join them on their journey through this landscape, walking with them as companions for at least a little part of their route? If we are to tolerate seemingly bizarre and often difficult behaviour we have to extend our understanding and increase our tolerance to their pain. A detailed knowledge of the person's past becomes the means by which we extend our capacity to venture, to explore, to remain a travelling companion for more of the journey and postpone for a time the parting of the ways.

So little is known about the world of the person with dementia. We should not assume that because what they express has no meaning for us, it has no meaning for them. People may be locked in to their own private worlds and the usual conversational conventions and our lack of skill forbid us gaining entry. The challenge is to find ways around the 'no entry' signs, to find new methods of communicating, new ways of relating.

The onus for initiating and sustaining conversation has to rest with the carer and for many this burden becomes too great. With the best intentions they try to conduct one sided conversations, and the very one sidedness means the conversation can not be sustained. It peters out, the carer feels a failure and isolation is compounded.

How is it possible to help significant members of the present social networks of people with dementia establish or sustain relationships which are to some extent reciprocal, rather than one-sided? The key is to understand past networks, the people, places and activities that used to be significant. If the life history of the person with dementia is known in considerable detail, this specific knowledge can be used as the basis on which to re-establish conversation. In this way the person's past is used to work for them in the present.

Reminiscence is one effective way to contribute to the complication of a life history. As Pear (1922) suggested, the mind paints pictures rather than takes photographs and so inaccuracies or inconsistencies over time in reminiscence are inevitable. Reminiscence is a natural process, often occurring spontaneously either in public or in private. It can, however, be deliberately evoked and purposely used for both general and specific social and therapeutic ends. Gibson (1989), Norris (1986) have outlined the various purposes and uses of reminiscence for both individuals and small groups.

When using reminiscence it is essential to set clear objectives. It is helpful to distinguish between spontaneous and planned reminiscence, individual and group work, reminiscence with people with dementia and people without dementia, and 'ordinary' and 'special' reminiscence work.

The skill level of workers and the context in which the reminiscence work is undertaken can have a crucial bearing on its nature and outcomes.

Either 'ordinary' or 'special' reminiscence may be undertaken with people with dementia. It may be used with either individuals or very small groups. Groups must be small, members carefully selected, and hyperactive, aggressive and emotionally liable people excluded. Multiple leaders or helpers who are familiar with the social background, accent and idiom of the group members can act as 'translators' or 'interpreters'. Multisensory triggers, particularly tangible artifacts and music which relate closely to the members' backgrounds and general interests are essential. Leaders need to be flexible, imaginative and responsive and the length of sessions should reflect the level of interest, attention and mood of the group.

All around multisensory triggers abound such as family photographs, letters, newspapers, books, magazines, familiar possessions and neighbourhoods where people live. All can be used to initiate conversation or to respond sensitively to some opening made by others. It is important to be finely tuned to the possibilities for spontaneous reminiscence, to understand its significance and potential for achieving mutually fruitful and often pleasurable change.

'Ordinary' reminiscence work can be a useful working tool for the many people with dementia who may not be preoccupied with aspects of their past, not particularly troubled in the present. When encouraged to talk about the past they derive obvious pleasure, albeit usually transitory. Those who share their pleasure and lucidity are so encouraged and intrigued that their behaviour towards the person with dementia can change radically. Reminiscence work gives pleasure, challenges endemic boredom and provides staff with abundant opportunities for their own personal and professional development.

Reminiscence work helps us use the then and there of life to enrich the here and now. It is widely accepted that reminiscence work has many valuable outcomes although it does not improve cognitive functioning. Positive outcomes as Fielden (1990), Bender (1989), Gibson (1989) and Kaminsky (1988), among others, have identified include increased sociability, improved general wellbeing characterised by improved appetite, decreased restlessness, reduction in challenging behaviours, lessened social isolation and improved mood.

Carers involved in reminiscence report increased interest in individuals and a growing ability to treat them as unique people. Increased tolerance of aberrant behaviour, and a willingness to be available to the older person and to share more closely in the pain of their lost abilities have also been reported. Staff find they can enter more fully into the reality and time frame of the person with dementia. Although never lying or deliberately seeking to mislead, they become less demanding about conformity to their own present reality of the time and place. Relatives have found increased tolerance, acceptance and a willingness to persevere in sustaining relationships.

There is of course continuing need for rigorous evaluative studies, as Thornton and Brotchie (1987) would attest. While this evidence is being accumulated, there is already enough known to justify encouraging social workers and other to use reminiscence which so evidently benefits older people, including people with dementia, their professional carers and family members.

HOW CAN THE PAST BE USED?

Using reminiscence work in a more focused, intensive and 'special' way with people with dementia whose behaviour is especially troubled and troublesome can achieve even more effective outcomes. To support this assertion several case studies gathered in the course of a small project will be cited. They summarise work undertaken in three statutory specialist homes for mentally infirm people and one specialist elderly community care team. The results from this project which involved intensive work with six individuals over eight months were so encouraging that it seems reasonable to suggest other residential and field social workers might profitably use a similar approach.

Senior managers in the homes were invited by a researcher/consultant to identify 'their most troublesome resident' and enable designated staff, 'keyworkers' to make special efforts with these identified people. Subsequently, a community care team adopted a similar approach.

Such investment of time in specific individuals was justified on two grounds. First, the troublesome individual is worthy of it in his/her own right. This is the idea of creative, rather than proportionate justice, a central principle adopted from Docker-Drysdale's (1968, 1973) work with disturbed children. Individualisation is now readily accepted as good child care practice where children are regarded as worthy of personalised idiosyncratic care. They are not all treated the same because their needs are not the same. Individualised care which is necessary for children is no less necessary for older people, especially for older people with dementia.

Second, if the troublesome behaviour of troubled residents can be reduced, life for all around them, both residents and staff will also be improved. This approach, which stresses treating people as unique individuals, is so ordinary that it hardly warrants attention, were it not for the pervasive therapeutic pessimism so characteristic of most contemporary social work practice with older people, and especially practice with older people with dementia.

The evaluation of the project's outcomes was based on careful recording of case studies. No rigorous investigation of outcomes was undertaken but the recorded observations of a number of different informants concerned with each case was used as the basis for drawing conclusions.

To provide a framework, eight stages in the work were identified and each worker was left free to proceed as best fitted their circumstances. Periodically, the key workers, line managers and the research/consultant met to plan, encourage, monitor and review.

1. Achieving the backing of management.

2. Identifying the person or subject.

3. Special observation.

4. Compiling a detailed life history.

5. Planning the special work.

6. Putting the plan into action.

7. Evaluating the work.

8. Continuing the work and generalising from it.

1. Achieving the backing of management
This was crucially important and it proved impossible to proceed effectively without it. Active, not passive support was essential. Senior staff needed to be responsible for explaining the nature of the 'special' work to the rest of their staff. Otherwise the burden was too great for any one

individual, the work was too isolated, lacked reinforcement and could be sabotaged in innumerable ways by others not committed to it.

For example:

> May, aged eighty, had been asked to leave six homes before coming to the present one. She was a poor eater, exceedingly hostile, prone to scratching and kicking, always verbally aggressive, extremely isolated and universally regarded as extremely difficult.

It was learned from her niece that Mary had always been fastidious about food and particular about its presentation. She liked 'nice things'. The staff brought her an attractive china cup, saucer and plate and her key worker who was determined to reduce Mary's isolation and improve her food intake would set a breakfast tray with a linen tray cloth, the special china and a small posy of flowers.

The first time the tray was presented, Mary, who rarely spoke except to swear, smiled, seemed pleased and said to the keyworker 'That's nice. You care about me.'

When the key worker was not on duty, the tray remained unset by the domestic staff who objected to a resident getting special attention. Finally the keyworker had to ask the matron to instruct the domestic staff to set the tray and not subvert the care plan.

2. Identifying the person or subject

Everyone, when asked to identify their most troublesome resident, could instantaneously do so. Those identified where people who were noisy, hostile, aggressive, disruptive, violent and non-conforming or else they were quiet, withdrawn people who the staff worried about because they realised they paid them so little personal attention.

3. Special observation

Two of the homes began their work with the discipline of observation. Simple proformas were used and all staff were able to share this stage of the work and to feel involved. The observations were taken over several days and throughout the 24 hour daily cycle to identify rhythms, patterns of recurring behaviours, or particular times of the day when the person might be especially troubled or disoriented.

Such a systematic approach to observed behaviour is not unlike Seed's use of diaries (1990) to study present networks. Behaviour in interaction with others and alone and the spatial locations in which these behaviours occurred were all recorded. The observations covered:

- Social interaction with residents, staff and others
- Behaviour – relevance and appropriateness
- Nature of speech – content and coherence, with whom, whether initiated or responsive
- Variations in lucidity, activity level and mood especially around key times of meals, bedtimes, bathing and toileting
- Personal likes – food, preferred space used for sitting and with whom
- Occupation, interests, domestic or other involvement
- Activities and capability concerned with self care
- Contacts – with family, friends, volunteers, others

Such observations told staff about the here and now life of the person and also gave them clues about other things, places, people and the past that they needed to inform themselves about.

4. Compiling a detailed life history

A detailed life history compiled by using all available informants and sources was central to this work. Knowledge of the person's past networks was important both in terms of providing leads to possible informants as well as uncovering information about crucial aspects of the person's life, interests, significant relationships and important places and events.

The person with dementia was used as a source of information. Staff were encouraged to believe them rather than disbelieve. Often conversations needed to be decoded but when staff began from the assumption of truth rather than falsity, belief rather than disbelief they made more progress. They tried to learn to decipher symbolic and coded communications and to respond to people's feelings. Unfortunately, workers did not always manage to do this. They were so conditioned to attributing confabulation and dismissing any reference to painful events as evidence of 'confusion', that they lost opportunities for history gathering and communication about past disturbing experiences. For example:

> Mary, who talked very little other than to swear, ('Go to hell' was her most common phrase), told the key worker she once had a baby

which did not live long. Her record showed her as childless so the worker decided the story was erroneous and so did not respond.

When asked, a relative corroborated the story. The worker had missed an opportunity to empathise and relate to a painful experience which had leaked into the present, even though it was a recollection of loss occurring more than fifty years before. Mary's attempt at communication was dismissed, a chance was lost to share the painful recollection and to show that she was understood.

The agency records almost always proved a disappointing source of information and were usually restricted to assessments of present functioning. Most of the residential records were extremely brief and superficial. These residents seemed more like displaced people, without a past, refugees in a strange and unfamiliar country whose whole long lives had been reduced to a few short lines.

Whenever possible, life history details were gathered from contemporary friends and relatives. They proved to be the best informants. By actually reminiscing with them, very comprehensive, detailed histories were gathered. Sometimes the person with dementia joined in these recall sessions. Details of chronological events, family life work, major life crises, landmarks and transitions, places where the person had lived and visited were all important. Reminiscence was the means used to compile a retrospective picture of past networks whereas direct observation of behaviour provided a contemporary picture. This dual approach was no mere sterile observation and social history taking but rather a means by which the rich colour and texture of a person's life could be sketched.

The fine-grained detail of the person's life was gathered. For example:

- Did the person like to have their hair permed?
- Did they like a hard or a soft pillow?
- Did they use an alarm clock?
- Were they interested in clothes?
- Did they like jewellery?
- Did they eat sliced or unsliced bread?
- What were their hobbies and interests?
- Were they houseproud?
- Who was their favourite film star?

- Where had they lived/worked/holidayed?
- Who had been their significant others?
- Who was still likely to be significant?

By putting other people's reminiscence to work on behalf of the person with dementia it is possible to gain access to information about the past which can then be used to improve their present. This reminiscence process can of itself prove helpful to relatives, especially their older spouses and friends who often feel included, shut our and unable to reach their loved one or help them in any effective way.

5. Planning the special work

By this time all the key workers had decided what 'special' interventions might be tried. They were encouraged to make a written plan but the plan was always regarded as flexible because such work needs to be planned yet spontaneous, to proceed moment by moment within a broad overall framework. The plan was regarded as a guide to a possible journey and if the journey took unexpected turns then the worker would seek to follow as best she could, being finely tuned to the present needs as well as the known past history.

It matters little whether such a written statement is called a goal plan (Barrowclough and Flemming 1986) or a care plan, providing it is ethical, relevant, practical, feasible and quite specific about the behaviour expected of the key worker and the complementary roles to be played consistently by other staff.

6. Putting the plan into action

Intervention began from the minute it was decided to do something; indeed, if it had been decided to do nothing, that too would have been intervention. Some of the intervention was tangible and rested on the implementation of agreed plans and activities, some of it was more intangible and involved staff's heightened curiosity and increased interest in the old person.

Detailed knowledge about past history identified people, places and pastimes which could be exploited in the present. Such knowledge made pilgrimages to past places of significance possible. It also made present involvement in particular pastimes richly gratifying.

For example:

> Joan, a quiet withdrawn woman, was taken by the key worker and a domestic with whom she had a tenuous relationship to visit her only surviving sibling in a nursing home. From reminiscing during the visit it was discovered that Joan used to be very interested in greyhound racing. A trip to a greyhound stadium was planned and both Joan and her key worker had a marvellous night at the dogs. The shared outing gave a focus for many later happy conversations.

For example:

> From reminiscing with Mary's niece the key worker discovered that Mary was so short sighted that the first thing she did on waking was to put her hand under the pillow to reach for her spectacles. Even though she had been in the home a year no one had realised she needed spectacles. Mary agreed to have an optician visit but when he called she refused to cooperate.
>
> Subsequently, glasses were obtained using an earlier prescription and although Mary refused to wear them she clearly stated her views about the kind in brown frames she used to have and would now prefer. She also surprised staff when she inquired about the arrangements for payment. The new glasses remained unused as far as was known but from time to time Mary was seen taking them out of their case to polish them.

7. Evaluating the work

In order for knowledge to grow and practice skills to be refined it is essential that such work be critically scrutinised and subjected to peer evaluation. Sometimes it may be helpful to use rating scales, other standardised instruments and independent observers. An ethnography and qualitative approach, as in this project, may yield richer if less rigorous results.

In the work reported here the following outcomes were identified:

For residents

It was necessary to withdraw one woman from the project because of physical illness.

The most consistent gain for the other five people, three in residential care and two in the community, was increased sociability even if shown in very small but important ways which the following excerpts from the records illustrate:

> Hitherto she has always sat alone in the little lounge and would chase anyone who came near, using very colourful language. Mr H was sitting in the room as well yesterday. He is a new, quiet resident. She let him sit on and did not shout. His daughter and son in law arrived to visit. I suggested they should go to his bedroom. 'It's all right, dear. Let them stay,' she said.

> Occasionally another resident will wander into her room. She doesn't shout at them now or hit out at them. She now lets the domestic clean her room without fuss and actually talks to her, initiating conversation and calling her back to continue talking.

It was, however, not all gain, as a subsequent record noted:

> On bad days she still sits looking at the floor. She will not come to the lounge. On good days she lifts her head and intermittently looks at people passing in the corridor. We have decided to turn her chair around so she can look out and see who is passing by.

> On Christmas day she wore her new outfit with pleasure but when Father Christmas intruded into her bedroom uninvited she quickly told him to go to hell.

> This woman was disturbed by 'ordinary' reminiscence. When shown a photograph of a butcher's shop in the same village where her father's haberdashery shop had been located she was not pleased. Spitting on the picture she said 'Sam Smith never was any good.' As the daughter of another shopkeeper it was impossible to know what past experience, if any, lay behind her vehement response.

For staff

It was possible to identify a number of consistent gains. All staff acknowledged their abysmal ignorance of the person as a person in terms of knowledge about their past life lived out in so many different places over so many years.

The search for the life history itself motivated staff as well as relatives. They became intrigued, excited, and determined to find out and then to use the information in conversation, outings, and in planning to follow up particular interests or pastimes. Because of its own intrinsic nature, the life history proved to be a powerfully motivating force for staff development. The staff became fascinated with the person's past, and quickly grasped the possibility of using the life history as a working tool. They found they could put history to work. In recovering the past, the present came alive.

Staff freely acknowledged that their preconceptions were challenged. They admitted they had consigned people to pigeon holes, made assumptions about them on the flimsiest of evidence and treated them in ways which they now recognised as self-fulfilling prophecies. Repeatedly, staff got the behaviour they anticipated. The person conformed to what was expected of then while their real pain and loss was either unrecognised, disregarded or dismissed.

For example:

> A woman from a working class area repeatedly kicked off her shoes as well as frequently trying to take off her clothes. Staff had labelled her 'the stripper'. They had been told she had worked in a mill so had decided she had been a wet spinner, hence the preference to bare feet. When the history was gathered, they discovered she had been a mill worker for only a short period. After marrying a skilled tradesman she lived a comfortable life, only recently returning to the working class area after her husband's death.

Staff found it was possible to rekindle acceptable social behaviour. They discovered that if they set up the person's physical and emotional environment or 'life space' to conform to their past experience, the person picked up the cues and behaved accordingly. People were able 'to pass themselves' very successfully when taken out to places or put in situations which evoked long established but rusty social skills which had been learned long ago.

The project exposed some of the shortcomings inherent in residential care, even 'good' residential care. It highlighted the advantages of trying wherever possible to keep people with dementia in familiar environments, enmeshed within established networks, as the fieldwork case studies illustrate.

Staff admitted that, although they were well intentioned, and meant to cause no ill to the people in their care, they found it difficult to withstand, or even continue to notice how institutional routines had taken over. Certain things were being done in certain ways, for no other reason than habit or tradition. Closer examination showed that often these routines actually exacerbated rather than ameliorated disturbed and disturbing behaviour.

This project helped staff to take a second look at residential practices they had been taking for granted. They proved to be open, self-critical and highly motivated to achieve change. Reminiscence work proved to be subversive in that it challenged preconceptions, altered relationships and questioned long established routines. Involvement in life history work and reminiscence inexorably demanded closer, more personal involvement between people with dementia and those who shared their lives either as informal or formal carers.

Staff were delighted to develop their own practice skills and to reconceptualise the nature of their jobs. No longer do they accept that providing good physical care, important as that is, should be their only interest. They have found that they can cope with exceedingly troubled and troublesome people. Instead of being dismissed with the customary 'Go to hell', they were told 'You care'. Instead of taking three care assistants to bath someone and cut her finger nails they were asked 'Would you give me a wash down, please?' Seeing someone who rejected most food on offer asking for a second helping of pudding, was rich reward indeed. What hurt beyond measure was to have a senior colleague, three months into the project, and after acknowledged reduction in challenging behaviours still ask 'Is it right to give one person special attention?'

The community care team used a similar approach and structured their work in the same systematic way. Two case studies are cited as further illustration of 'special' reminiscence work.

Andy, aged sixty five, lived with his wife in the family home in an old, stable, suburban community. His three married children, two daughters and a son, lived nearby and visited frequently. In 1990 Andy was diagnosed as having early onset Alzheimer's disease and was referred by the psychogeriatrician to the specialist elderly community care team for day care assessment. At this time he retained good skills and was still talking to the various members of his social network.

Day care for two days each week was arranged to give him greater social stimulation and his wife time for housework, shopping and family visiting. In the two years after the referral he rapidly deteriorated, as assessed by Cape scores. During the first few months following the referral he became restless, agitated and increasingly withdrawn. From being a friendly, sociable man he became morose, totally silent, not even talking to his wife.

The explicit objective set by the social worker was to use life history information to try to re-establish communication between Andy and key people in his current network.

His health and social services network included a general practitioner, psychogeriatrician, day care workers and a field social worker. The latter encouraged the wife to observe meticulously and record in detail her husband's behaviour over a 48 hour period. The social worker compiled a detailed life history, taking ten year intervals to provide a structure and using the very willing wife as informant. This was done over several weeks during the time Andy was at the day centre. Specific information was gathered about his family of origin, childhood, school, courtship and marriage, residence in Australia, naval service, other work, significant family events and key people. This approach has much in common with Myer's (1991) and Ryan and Walker's (1985) use of life story books.

Andy's wife greatly enjoyed the social worker's undivided attention. She believed she was doing something positive to help her husband. Her reminiscing, in effect a life review, proved to be a positive experience for her and helped her value and affirm the long life she and Andy had shared together.

Close observation identified a recurring patter of acute restlessness and agitation in the early afternoons. Andy's life-long interest in classical guitar music was unearthed through the life history. Music provided a means of imaginative intervention. He could no longer manage to play the guitar himself but the social worker found he responded well to recorded guitar music. Each day after lunch his wife would put on a record, Andy would settle back in his favourite arm chair, close his eyes and listen attentively for up to an hour. His restless period was replaced by calm enjoyment – a gain for both himself and his wife.

The social worker also spent time with Andy in the day centre where she used the details of his life, gleaned from the wife's reminiscences, to introduce conversation about past times and events with which she was now familiar. Instead of conveying a vague general interest, she was able to be focused and specific in her conversation. She used a well ordered collection of family photographs and found Andy could sustain a largely lucid conversation despite his increasing deterioration.

He could not name people in the photographs but apparently recognised them, being able to recount events connected with the photographs. For example, when shown a family snap taken at Niagara Falls he recounted a long story about a woman who had thrown her baby over the Falls. The social worker reacted initially by thinking Andy's account of such a bizarre event must be confabulation. His wife later confirmed her husband's account in every detail.

The social worker considered she achieved reasonable success in reestablishing communication with Andy and between Andy and significant others in his network. Her overall time commitment was not increased but, by becoming more focused, her work became more effective. Andy appeared to enjoy his renewed exchange with people, his wife was able to contribute constructively to his care and his troublesome behaviour was reduced.

Dementia has taken its toll. Andy is now dead but, while he lived, his past was used to help ameliorate the ravages of the present.

Anabel, aged eighty five, was referred to the same social services team for domiciliary care assessment by the hospital where she was receiving treatment for a chest infection. She had a rich social network. Her supportive family lived near her sheltered dwelling, which was in the same inner city neighbourhood where she had spent her life. Her relatives called daily but because of their work were unable to make her a mid-day meal.

The social work assistant responding for the home help service interviewed the daughters who said their mother had left school early, married young, had ten children, only three of whom survived. Prior to her illness she had been house proud, fastidious, active and independent. They described their mother as a 'very private person' who had gradually become restless, demanding, difficult and neglectful of personal and domestic hygiene.

Initially, Anabel would scarcely speak to the social work assistant other than to make it very plain that she intended to remain in her own home. She would contemplate neither residential care nor day care.

In order to test whether she could accept a domiciliary worker coming into her house, which was considered to be the minimal service which might sustain her wish to remain at home, it was decided to use reminiscence to try to reach into her isolation and improve her communication. A detailed life history was gathered from various sources. Anabel herself and her daughters provided information about the family. The neighbourhood context was studied using the local library and other local contacts as resources. In these ways the social work assistant was able to place herself within the changing geographic and social context in which Anabel still lived.

Specific details about personal likes, dislikes, life style and preferences added colour. These details confirmed that Anabel, who all her life had kept herself to herself, could not and should not be expected, in late life to take on group activities or group living.

The history highlighted her past competence as the financial manager of the family, despite her limited education and her life-long interest in shopping, fashion, clothes and hairstyles.

This information was used to compile several tailor-made packages of reminiscence triggers especially for Anabel. Instead of using the widely available general reminiscence packs, the trigger material was specifically designed in order to increase its relevance and heighten its appeal. Packs on money and shopping, fashion, family life, anniversaries, reaction and current events were made. Triggers included photographs of the locality as it used to be, family photographs, old money, fashion catalogues and other artifacts such as clothing and footwear. Even a relevant trigger word, 'gusset boots' was guaranteed to catch Anabel's attention and make two-way conversation possible.

The packs were left in Anabel's house so that her daughters, home help, social work assistant or area warden could use them to catch her attention and focus conversation. She proved able, when appropriately stimulated, to respond with animation, interest and a fair degree of accuracy. She could sustain a conversation for several minutes but she could not initiate one.

Anabel's callers and carers felt better as their conversations were no longer one-sided. Because their social contact was more rewarding they were more likely to sustain visiting and caring, which means Anabel's wishes have been respected and, so far, she has been able to remain at home.

WHAT ARE THE IMPLICATIONS FOR SOCIAL WORK PRACTICE OF USING THE PAST?

Both 'ordinary' and 'special' reminiscence work can be beneficial for people with dementia. It may also help their family, friends and professional carers to sustain communication and gain more satisfaction from their relationships.

Such work uses what belongs to the person – their past – in their own service. The careful, specific, skilled use of the past seeks to promote or at least sustain for as long as possible, the person's independence.

As more people live into late old age, the number of very old people with cognitive impairment is liable to increase. More of them will be managed in the community. Those who eventually enter residential homes or nursing homes are likely to be the most seriously impaired and the most behaviourally disturbed, or be people with non-existent or impoverished social networks. There is, therefore, an urgent need to train skilled specialist staff who can be used as resources to support less experienced staff in day care, residential and nursing establishments, domiciliary staff and family carers in the community.

'Ordinary' reminiscence work should become a mainstream activity for everyone of any age whom might find it helpful. 'Special' reminiscence work should be tried with those more troubled people whose aberrant behaviour makes their humane management and care particularly challenging.

Involvement of significant others in the mutual process of reminiscence can help to re-establish shrinking social networks. Through some of the means which have been described, the person with dementia may be helped to sustain, or actually be reintroduced to social networks through involvement with others in either one-to-one work or very small reminiscence groups.

Shrinking networks almost always occur in late life. When dementia is added to the normative hazards of repeated loss in late life which includes the loss of significant others, places, possessions and capacities, shrinkage of networks is bound to be accelerated. Using the past can be a way of retarding this almost inexorable process.

By using knowledge about past networks, present networks may be sustained. The future for people with dementia is usually bleak, although the rate of decline can be extremely variable. Thus all the person can be sure of is the present and the present needs to be made as rich and non-threatening as possible. The sensitive use of the past is one way of caring for them and also enriching their contemporary carers.

The worker has the responsibility to inform themselves, to locate the conversation within territory which is likely to be safe because it is familiar, and to avoid setting people up for failure. In valuing their past the worker is valuing them.

All life history and reminiscence work requires time. Where people with dementia are already receiving a service, it means a different, more productive use of time. People have to be attended to as unique individuals. Their need for personal recognition and respect is in no way diminished. Their need for close, warm, personal, unconditional regard may indeed be greater, rather than less because of their dementia.

Instead of being seen only as they are in the present as cognitively impaired, deteriorated and probably difficult, through reminiscence and life history work the individual's carer's sympathies may be enlarged and their patience extended. By sensitively using the past, the encroaching private worlds inhabited by people with dementia can be shared with others to a much greater degree than is otherwise possible.

This work requires good basic inter-personal skills of observation, reading verbal and non-verbal cues, attending, careful listening, responding and empathising as well as skills of data collection, recording and assessment. Being able to work with individuals, families and small groups is also necessary.

Social workers' understanding about dementia needs to grow more sophisticated. We need to relinquish popular global negative terms like 'living death', 'changed personalities' and 'lost people'. These generalities excuse us from the demanding and disciplined work of using life history. Universal negativism and therapeutic nihilism deter us from the fascinating search for the islands of lucidity. If we fail to locate the lucid, still intact parts of the person's memory, we may from their history at least get an inkling of what they are trying to communicate. We may better understand the garbled story and the confused statement. From our detailed knowledge we may know to what they are referring and then we may be better able to respond to the underlying emotion and intended communication.

The onus for initiating conversation needs to rest firmly with the carers. If the stimulus used is sufficiently relevant, conversations do not need to be one sided. By attitudes, behaviour and speech, the carer must reduce the sense of threat. The person with dementia must not fear that if she speaks she will be found out and her deficiencies disclosed. The conversation must be set within safe territory and familiar bounds.

This work demands that both professional and family carers be prepared to accept their own fears of being overwhelmed by another's pain. They must be willing to enter to some extent into the other's world. They must learn to value small gains, brief encounters, transitory happiness and fleeting rationality.

For a social worker or other professional carer to persuade themselves that their work is done when they have made an assessment, attached a diagnostic label, provided good quality physical care in a safe environment is to miss the excitement and the satisfaction inherent in using a person's past to work for them in the present.

Social workers and others must take the time to find ways of talking and ways of listening. They must be able to help network members, especially family carers, understand that although much is lost, some things remain. For many people, what remains may be able to be used to help rather than hinder, to include, rather than exclude, to encourage social interaction and decrease social isolation. In understanding the past, the present may be managed better and future threat contained or retarded.

REFERENCES

Barrowclough, C. and Flemming, I. (1986) *Goal Planning with Elderly People*. Manchester: Manchester University Press.

Bender, M.P. (1989) *Reminiscence Groupworkers: The Quiet Revolutionaries*. PSIGE Newsletter, 31, 20–24.

Bowlby, J. (1973) *Attachment and Loss, vol 2, Separation, Anxiety and Anger*. London: Hogarth.

Crawford, J., Kippax, S., Onyx, J. and Gault, U. (1990) Women Theorising their Experiences of Anger: a study using memory work. *Australian Psychologist*, 25. 3. 33–350.

Disch, R. (ed) (1988) *Twenty Five Years of the Life Review: Theoretical and Practical Considerations*. New York: Haworth.

Docker-Drysdale, B. (1968) *Therapy in Child Care Collected Papers*. Harlow: Longmans.

Docker-Drysdale, B. (1973) Consultation in Child Care *Collected Papers*. Harlow: Longmans.

Epstein, H. (1980) *Children of the Holocaust: Conversations with Sons and Daughters of Survivors*. New York: Bantam.

Epstein, E.R. and Mendelsohn, R. (1978) *Record and Remember: Tracing Your Roots Through Oral History*. New York: Sovereign.

Fielden, M. (1990) Reminiscence as a therapeutic intervention with sheltered housing residents: a comparative study. *British Journal of Social Work*, 20, 1.

Gibson, F. (1989) *Using Reminiscence: Training Pack*. London: Help the Aged.

Haley, A. (1977) *Roots*. London: Hutchinson.

Harre, R. (1983) *Personal Being*. Oxford: Blackwell.

Haugh, F. (1987) *Female Sexualization*. London: Verso.

Hewitt, J. (1942) Once alien here. In J. Hewitt and J. Montague (1970) *The Planter and the Gael*. Belfast: Arts Council.

Kaminsky, M. (1988) All that our eyes have witnessed: memories of a living workshop in the South Brons. In R. Disch *Twenty Five Years of the Life Review*. New York: Haworth.

McWhenney, A. (1967) *Adopted Children and How They Grow Up*. London: Routledge.

Miesen, B. (1992) Attachment Theory and Dementia. In G. Jones and B. Miesen (ed) *Care-Giving in Dementia*. London: Tavistock.

Molinari, V. and Reichlin, R.E. (1984) Life review reminiscence in the elderly: a review of the literature. *International Journal of Aging and Human Development* 20, 2, 81–93.

Morgan, S. (1991) *My Place*. London: Virago.

Myers, K. (1991) *Life Story Books*. Stirling: Dementia Services Development Centre.

Norris, A. (1986) *Reminiscence With Elderly People*. Bicester: Winslow.

Pear, T.H. (1922) *Remembering and Forgetting*. London: Methuen.

Ryan, T. and Walker, R. (1985) *Making Life Story Books*. London: BAAF.

Seed, P. (1990) *Introducing Network Analysis in Social Work*. London: Jessica Kingsley Publishers.

Tarman, V.I. (1988) Autobiography: the negotiation of a lifetime. *International Journal of Aging and Human Development* 27, 3, 171–191.

Thornton, S. and Brotchie, J. (1987) Reminiscence: a critical review of the literature. *British Journal of Clinical Psychology* 26, 93–111.

Triseliotis, J. (1973) *In Search of Origins*. London: Routledge.

POINTS FOR DISCUSSION

1. Does your own experience in working with people with dementia confirm the statement: 'A detailed knowledge of the person's past becomes the means by which we extend our capacity to venture, to explore, to remain a travelling companion for more of the journey and postpone for a time the parting of the ways'.

2. Discuss the proposition that the key to sustain reciprocal relationships within current networks of people with dementia lies in understanding their past networks.

3. What is the difference between planned and spontaneous reminiscence and in what ways is reminiscence initiated and managed?

4. Consider the use of information about current and past social networks to help people with dementia like Mary and Jane who needed special reminiscence work in a residential setting. On what grounds is such 'special work' justified? How are the benefits evaluated?

5. With particular reference to the examples of Andy and Anabel, discuss the proposition that life history and reminiscence work using a social network approach mean that 'people have to be attended to as unique individuals'. How would people with dementia otherwise tend to be regarded?

CHAPTER FOUR

Systemic Family Intervention

Joanne Sherlock and Iain Gardner

INTRODUCTION

For social workers, the concept of intervening with a family as the client is not a new one. Historically, social work has taken a psychosocial approach to the way in which clients are viewed and most training in the field is underpinned by a systems model. As such, most clients of social work would be viewed a part of a family system, and in fact as part of the much wider social system.

Dementia is an illness which generally impacts on the whole family and it is therefore valuable for workers in this field to develop skills in intervening with the family as a unit.

This chapter outlines some of the skills of intervention which may be useful when working with families where dementia is present. It must be stressed that it is essential that, before attempting to implement any family intervention, workers should have a solid knowledge of and practised supervision in the basic counselling skills.

FAMILY THERAPY AND FAMILY INTERVENTION

Family therapy is practised by a wide range of professionals in a variety of settings. It is firmly underpinned by General Systems Theory which also underpins much of social work practice. Systems theory is not a method of working but provides global concepts that are relevant to understanding the dynamic nature of all living organisms. It provides the worker with a way of viewing personal and social situations in the context in which they occur. It can be viewed as a paradigm which enables the worker to view an individual as a member of a family system. The family system is then viewed in the context of other systems within society.

Workers typically encounter family systems when they are under stress and their focus is on identifying problems and attempting to resolve conflict in order to enhance its functioning as a system. The main focus from a systems view is to locate the boundaries, not only between the family and the environment, but also between the subsystems. The worker assesses the degree of openness and closeness of the system and the relationship and communication patterns that exist.

Family therapy aims to change existing relationships within a family so that the symptomatic behaviour disappears. It is an attempt to modify family relationships to achieve harmony. The family is acknowledged as being a vital source of development, influence and assistance to individuals within the family system but is also considered to have the ability to generate stress and to cause dysfunction.

One of the underpinning principles of family therapy is the concept of homeostasis. That is, within any family system a state of equilibrium will be maintained. If a problem exists in one part of the system then it is most likely to influence the whole family and will need to be accommodated by other family members. Likewise, any positive changes within one part of the family will influence and need to be accommodated by the rest of the system.

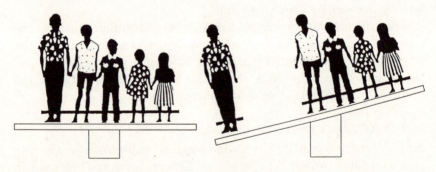

A: Family in balance   B: Family require readjustment

Figure 4.1 Equilibrium in the Family

The emphasis of the family therapy process is on harnessing the dynamics of the family system to bring about change which leads to harmony. The therapist enters the family system, which by and of itself is a powerful part of the process. In observing how the family accommodates the therapist, much is learnt about how the family functions or dysfunctions. Having entered into the family system the therapist endeavours to assist the family to learn about their current functioning and to discover new and more functional ways of coping with problems. The therapist guides and challenges the family to develop new perceptions of their system and to establish new ways of interacting which lead to a more satisfying and harmonious lifestyle.

Family therapy can be viewed in two distinct and separate ways. In its original form it can be viewed as a Modality of Practice where all family members were seen simultaneously and the basis of the therapeutic process and the mode of treatment was the family process itself. Over the years of its development this purest approach has been modified to accommodate working with individuals and subgroups of the family system. There are a variety of styles of family therapy which fall into this category and they can be investigated further by exploring the suggested reading at the end of the chapter.

Another way of viewing family therapy is as an orientation to practice. This is a psychosocial viewpoint whereby it is acknowledged that the family is a significant determinant of personality development and social behaviour and it is therefore necessary for workers to have an under-standing of it and to consider the family when working with any client. It does not necessarily imply that all therapy will be provided in the family setting but rather implies the importance of the family to the individual in contributing to therapeutic change.

It is in fact a systemic approach to intervention with individuals and families rather than family therapy in its purest, traditional form. It is this view of family therapy as an orientation to practise which is discussed in this chapter as the most applicable approach to dealing with families where dementia is present.

In looking at modern family therapists *The Networker* (1988) reported on some interesting statistics from their research. Figure 4.2 outlines the statistics of the average age and family position of therapists, length of treatment, caseload characteristics and theoretical orientations. This in-formation reinforces the relatively short-term nature of the intervention,

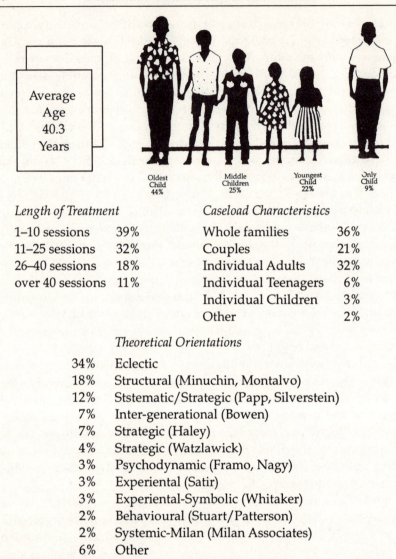

Average
Age
40.3
Years

Oldest
Child
44%

Middle
Children
25%

Youngest
Child
22%

Only
Child
9%

Length of Treatment

1–10 sessions	39%
11–25 sessions	32%
26–40 sessions	18%
over 40 sessions	11%

Caseload Characteristics

Whole families	36%
Couples	21%
Individual Adults	32%
Individual Teenagers	6%
Individual Children	3%
Other	2%

Theoretical Orientations

34%	Eclectic
18%	Structural (Minuchin, Montalvo)
12%	Ststematic/Strategic (Papp, Silverstein)
7%	Inter-generational (Bowen)
7%	Strategic (Haley)
4%	Strategic (Watzlawick)
3%	Psychodynamic (Framo, Nagy)
3%	Experiental (Satir)
3%	Experiental-Symbolic (Whitaker)
2%	Behavioural (Stuart/Patterson)
2%	Systemic-Milan (Milan Associates)
6%	Other

Figure 4.2: Family Therapist Survey Results. The Networker Jan/Feb 1988

the spread of family members seen and the many different approaches. Perhaps the most interesting finding is that 34 per cent of therapists are eclectic in their approach. That is, they use a variety of approaches as appropriate to their client's needs. This is a view that the authors support in dealing with families where dementia is present. Workers should develop a range of skills from which they can choose the most appropriate according to the varied needs of their clients.

In providing care to a person with dementia there are many decisions that have to be made by families. Most of the problems encountered by families are complex, multifaceted, and involve a variety of possible options to choose from. These problems are often new to the family so the decisions have to be made outside an existing comfort zone. This need to make decisions for someone else, particularly under stress, has great potential to generate conflict within families. It is likely that within any one family there will be a variety of ideas, theories and values about what is the best solution, and even although each member might be acting with the best intention, there is often not one right way to solve the problem. This is often the time when unresolved conflicts from the past reappear and influence the decision making process. It is not unreasonable to expect that, even in the healthiest families, there will be a degree of unresolved conflict just waiting for the opportunity to surface. Family intervention can confront this conflict head on by assisting families to identify its causes and to reach agreement about how best they can deal with it. It must be remembered that if conflict is dealt with constructively it results in better decisions being made. So the families that do not acknowledge their conflict can often be just as dysfunctional, if not more so than those who appear to be in constant conflict situations.

The dementia process generates stress which in turn can bring families into a dysfunctional state. However, the stress by and of itself can result in dysfunction. Individuals experience a primary stress response to stressors which can be seen to have a parallel process with a stress response in the family. Stress, if not dealt with, will have disastrous, physical and psychological effects on the family. It is essential that families find creative and constructive ways in which to deal with their stress. These issues lend themselves very nicely to being dealt with in family sessions.

Depression is also part of the dementia process. The person with dementia often suffers depression as a symptom of neurological degeneration and also as a reaction to having a chronic illness. Similarly, the family members, both individually and collectively, may display symptoms of depression. If the family as a whole is depressed then it is unlikely that it will remain functional. The objective becomes to optimize the family's functioning to enable them to meet their individual and shared objectives and needs.

The systemic family intervention approach has much to offer families where dementia is present. There is a need to reduce the stress in the family and to enhance the functioning of the family. The family approach can assist families by increasing their awareness about their current dynamics and functioning and by exploring alternate ways for them to frame issues, relate to each other and to solve problems creatively.

INDICATORS FOR FAMILY INTERVENTION
WHERE DEMENTIA IS PRESENT

It is difficult to be too specific about when the systemic family approach should be used and when it should not. Workers who lean more towards a systems framework would be more likely to see most psychosocial problems as being appropriately dealt with by this approach. Nevertheless, regardless of the worker's orientation, there are some indicators with families where dementia is present which suggest that this approach should be taken. They include:

- families in crisis
- conflict situations
- changing roles and relationships
- symptoms of depression
- prolonged dysfunctioning
- sexual issues
- behaviour problems
- symptoms of stress
- confusion

It is necessary to have the support of the family. The initial task of the worker is to assist the family in identifying what the problem is and what objectives they have for the intervention.

CONCEPTS AND PROCESSES

Most clients are in a distressed state when they seek help. It is important then that they have a sense of change reasonably promptly. This is most appropriately achieved by:

- gathering essential psychosocial details
- clarifying the family's experience to date
- determining what it is the family wants; whether that is:
  - ○ practical advice (behaviour management strategies)
  - ○ links to local resources and carer support groups
  - ○ therapy in relation to their role as a member of a family in which dementia is present

If the individual and/or the family want to engage in therapy, the following is an outline of aspects involved in that process.

The Family Assessment Wheel

A helpful tool in clarifying the client's current state of functioning, their expectations of therapy and how they will know that they have achieved what they want, is by assessment and then a mutually agreed upon contract between the client and the worker. Together they can look at the client's current and past abilities, strengths and functioning patterns. By working through the various segments of the Family Assessment Wheel, (Figure 4.3) both parties will develop a strong base from which therapy can proceed. This will also indicate a framework for therapy and allow both client and worker the opportunity to establish their respective boundaries. The contract can be periodically reviewed as therapy progresses. This is helpful as it keeps the process on track and evolving.

The Family Assessment Wheel attempts to bring together many of the influencing factors that impact on individual and family functioning. Emotionally we are made up of a variety of experiences taken from a broad spectrum of influences. The Family Assessment Wheel is only a guide and it is not necessary to gather information from each and every segment if it is not appropriate. It is hoped the Family Assessment Wheel will assist workers with the task of assessment. By asking questions that incorporate the Who? Which? Why? Where? and How? of each section, a clearer picture of family functioning will become apparent to client and worker alike.

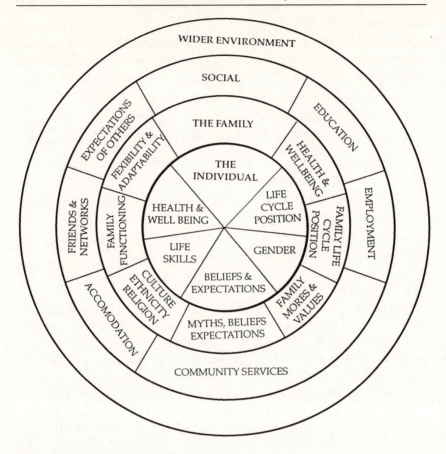

Figure 4.3: The Family Assessment Wheel

The use of an assessment tool such as the Family Assessment Wheel will draw out information about individual and family beliefs and mores that the client may or may not be consciously aware of but which nevertheless affect their day to day life. For example, a client may see herself as functioning in isolation and judge her ability to be an effective carer as such, without considering the other daily living pressures that are impinging upon her. The system she lives in may make it impossible for her to feel successful in her role as carer. A family message, whether explicit or implicit, may be: 'We do not allow people who are not family members to help us'. Thus the message from her family is 'You are not successful because you can not manage alone'. The aim of therapy would be to explore, eventually challenge, and ultimately reframe it into a more constructive belief; one that contributes to healthy carer functioning and allows the client the opportunity to seek the assistance she truly believes will help her.

By evaluating the various aspects of the Family Assessment Wheel, and how this impacts on individual and family functioning, we develop a far more systemic picture. Assessment of current functioning assists the therapeutic relationship by indicating probable areas that need to be considered. As part of the assessment process, both parties can also begin to consider how the therapeutic process can be put into action.

A thorough assessment will establish a strong base upon which the therapy can proceed. Typically, assessment involves defining with the client, and mutually arriving at guidelines for therapy. A contract will then define the boundaries within which therapy is to occur. Some important aspects of assessment that need to be covered are as follows.

It is essential to determine why it is the client has come to see you and what it is they seek assistance with. Equally important is to clarify why it is now that they are looking for help; what has changed; and what their experience has been to date. (What has been occurring in their life, and the person with dementia's life.) Also, what previous involvement and experience of therapy have they had? Exploring the solutions they have found to date in dealing with the presenting issue(s) is also appropriate at this point. In covering the above outlined basics, the immediate future direction will be established. For instance, as an extreme example, if it is apparent that the carer can no longer cope and the person with dementia is at risk, then a crisis intervention mode would be the most appropriate course of action.

Contracts

A more likely scenario will be one where the worker and client envisage similar issues to be addressed. It is then necessary to enter into a contract for therapy. A contract can be formal, as in a signed statement, or simply an informal verbal agreement. Contracts are a constant reminder as to why we meet with people and a valuable yardstick by which to evaluate the therapy process. Contracting requires both client and worker mutually to decide why they are meeting and also how they will know they have achieved what it is they wish to achieve. For example, it clarifies the client's belief about what will be achieved by therapy – whether these are realistic beliefs or fantasy based: 'This person (the therapist) will fix it up for me'. The more concrete and specific the contract guidelines are, the better the possibility of achievement. Clear guidelines will also facilitate a straightforward evaluation of the therapy process.

Contracts also incorporate any financial contributions involved, and if appropriate *an explanation regarding worker obligations and mandatory reporting in the likelihood of elder abuse.* Agency expectations of the worker regarding limitations on the number of therapy sessions; if the assessment is part of an intake interview informing the client that they may have to go on a waiting list, or if they will be seeing another worker. (If this is the case the subsequent worker would then re-contract with the client.) Contracts also include agreements on how frequently and over what time-frame people will need, for example, one hourly session every second week for two months.

The intervention process is part of the client assessment and client/worker contract. For the purposes of explanation the three have been separated but in reality they are mutually dependent and interconnected. For example, circular questions are a helpful tool to use during the assessment process and also at any stage throughout therapy. Most frequently people seek assistance due to their own stress and the distress of dealing with a chronic degenerative illness – their ambivalence at being 'caught' in such a difficult and demanding role, and their need to redress the expectation of the wider system that they should provide care to a person with dementia.

A number of different skills can be used to assist the individual/family to develop an understanding of the impact their world view is having on their everyday functioning. The process involved in family intervention varies from one individual/family to the next. Everyone has different strengths and abilities and consequently act and react differently.

CASE EXAMPLE

June presented in a very distressed state. Her parents had recently gone into sheltered care. Her father had severe arthritis as well as a recent hospital admission for cancer of the prostate. Her mother was in stage two of Alzheimer's disease. They were no longer able to manage at home as their health needs had deteriorated to such an extent that they needed constant supervision and support. June had coped quite well with arranging Geriatric Assessment Team involvement and in facilitating sheltered care admission. Her problem as she defined it was with her younger sister and their interaction about their parents.

It would seem that one way of addressing these concerns would be to invite the sister in to discuss the situation further. June was not able to consider this as she felt her sister to be too overpowering.

Dilemmas such as these can lead the therapist to believe that unless the sister attends also, not much can be achieved. This is not accurate. The process of family intervention and skills used are not restricted to numbers of people. Information about those who cannot be present physically can be obtained. The use of circular questioning is one method of doing this.

Circular questioning

Circular questioning is a style credited to the Milan Group of Family Therapists. The aim of circular questioning is to gather information about behaviour(s) that occur around the disease/illness. It has been likened to asking family members to 'gossip' about one another. The therapist asks the client how they believe another family member would respond to a given situation. The other main feature is that circular questioning highlights differences between family members in their response to situations. The concepts of circularity are readily grasped but require considerable practice and expertise to be used effectively in therapy.

Genograms

Genograms also form a valuable diagrammatic presentation of family structure (Figure 4.4). Usually they are drawn with information from three generations – current, family of origin and grandparents, but may include other generations if the information is available. Using genograms in the assessment process contributes to the information gathering. Often clients have not seen their family depicted in such a way before and they become aware of strong themes and similarities. Writing details on the genogram concerning individual members increases client and worker awareness.

Multigenerational beliefs of ageing and what it means to grow old will become apparent. For example, if it has been the experience of older members within a family that being old is a natural and normal part of

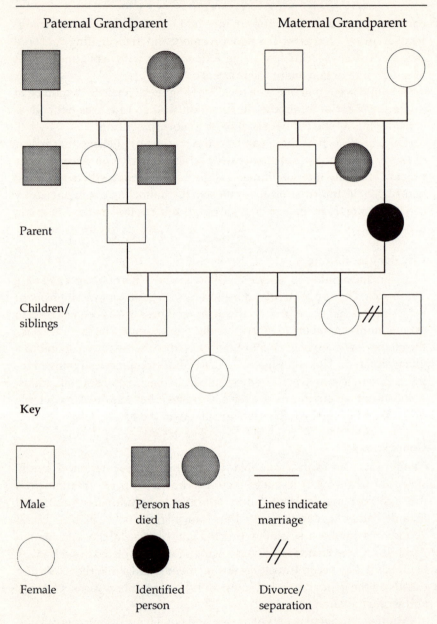

Paternal Grandparent   Maternal Grandparent

Parent

Children/
siblings

Key

Male

Person has
died

Lines indicate
marriage

Female

Identified
person

Divorce/
separation

Source: Genograms in family assessment, McGoldrick and Gerson 1985
Figure 4.4: Genogram: Diagram of a family over three generations

life's processes and that there is still much to be learned, subsequent generations will also have a positive outlook on ageing. If the family has not experienced either chronic illness within its ranks before, or they have had little or no contact with older people it is likely they will be highly anxious and not have developed adequate and appropriate coping skills.

Genograms are also a useful subjective means of recording anecdotal data on family illness and disease. This is particularly relevant as regards dementia as it is only in recent years that it has been acknowledged as a disease rather than an inevitable part of ageing. By recording this data the worker will add to the growing world-wide statistical information on dementia.

The symbols used to depict the various generations, sex of family members, marriage lines, order of birth, and so forth are all standardised. Further information on genograms can be obtained by consulting the recommended reading list at the end of this chapter.

Sculpting

Another skill that can assist the family by developing their awareness is sculpting. Sculpting is an interactive participatory process in which the family, with support and direction from the worker, depicts their emotional connectedness and feelings and impressions of and toward one another. For example, a family member may feel distanced and cut off from their family and may choose to indicate this by being as far from the remainder of the family as they can, within the limitations of the room in which sculpting occurs.

Sculpting is a family intervention skill that is not recommended for use by the novice. Sculpting has the potential to be extremely powerful and ought not be attempted by those lacking the training and experience to address the issues raised in a therapy session in which sculpting is used. Other more widely practised skills are the prescription of homework for the individual or family, behaviour modification and problem solving skills.

Homework

The prescription of homework is designed to encourage the family to practice the changes they have spoken of in therapy. As part of the assessment and therapeutic process the clients will have highlighted issues that they wish to resolve. They will also have gained knowledge as to how they are contributing to the maintenance of the problem; that is, the role they play in producing it. Homework encourages families to practice new ways of interacting. It also establishes guidelines for the context in which homework is to occur. For example, if the primary carer is feeling unsupported by the other family members she may need to state 'I am feeling unsupported, and would like some help with dressing Grandmother'. Often family members want to help but are unsure how to provide this assistance.

Methods of dealing with problem behaviour

The disease process of dementia can also manifest problem behaviours in people with dementia. As a worker it is important to help families develop strategies to deal with what are often socially embarrassing, demanding and sometimes threatening behaviours. Helping them to solve problems creatively will often alleviate the situation. For example, if the person with dementia becomes agitated at bath time, analyse the interaction that takes place. Asking questions such as who is involved? What in particular are they objecting to? Is it the person who is requesting they take a bath? Are they feeling insecure? Is it necessary for them to bath at this time? For whose benefit is it: the carer or the person with dementia? Is the bathroom warm enough? Does the person feel unsure because they find the situation threatening in some way? And so forth.

By gathering practical tips and anecdotal information, the worker can use such information to assist the carer to feel they are not alone in their struggle and may also help them with a solution to their problem. An example that comes to mind is helping carers deal with the vexing question of when the person with dementia should no longer drive and how this can be most diplomatically approached.

Many of the problem solving skills and behaviour modification strategies have been borrowed from the psychiatric care field, and adapted for application with a person with dementia. It is to the original source that workers should return for further reading.

Evaluation

The evaluation of the family intervention process will be assisted by the initial assessment and the subsequent contract agreement. Throughout therapy it is worthwhile to return to the contract (a written contract is far more helpful for this process). By re-evaluating the various steps and guidelines and reviewing the appropriateness for them, a positive outcome in terms of the objectives will be assured. The clearer and more concrete the objectives the more likely the client will have their needs met through the therapy process.

To conclude, a systemic approach to family intervention is a valuable and appropriate means of assisting families to cope better with caring for a person with dementia. A systemic approach assists by teasing out the threads of the carer's life and the role the person with dementia has had in it. We have attempted to outline some approaches borrowed from family therapy that are most appropriate and helpful to families dealing with a chronic and degenerative illness such as dementia.

WORKER ISSUES

Care giving is a gender issue. By far the majority of carers are women: wives, mothers, daughters, sisters, daughters-in-law. Often they combine a caring role with other roles and responsibilities, frequently giving up paid employment to become a full-time unpaid carer. Financial compensation in the form of a carer's pension and so forth is inadequate. This is particularly so when compared to the financial cost of institutional care.

As workers we can contribute to the rebalance of this inequity by being pro-active in the push for better and more appropriate services. Women, too, need to reflect on the role they play in continuing to maintain the *status quo*. Many carers who are no longer involved in the day-to-day care and responsibility of a person with dementia are able to band together to agitate and lobby government for a better choice in services for people with dementia and their carers. Carers whose life situations are such that their energies are channelled toward the care of people with dementia can be represented by workers. It is only by improving services to allow carers a true choice that change will occur. Choice will allow carers valuable respite and time to live a life of their own, independent of their role as carer.

A theme which perhaps has come through in this chapter is the need for workers to be generic in their approach. Drawing on a variety of therapeutic skills will assist the worker to maintain a client-centred approach with the end result that the client is more likely to receive what they need rather than what the worker believes they need. Carers of people with dementia are the experts. No one knows nor understands the person with dementia as well as they do. Many workers risk invalidating their clients by failing to work with and for them. For example, by allowing our own judgements or beliefs about how therapy ought to be progressing we attend to our own hidden agendas and not to the needs of our clients. It is therefore important for us as workers/therapists to monitor our reactions and judgements in order to minimise any possible negative outcome. Often simply acknowledging our reactions without judging ourselves, and putting them aside to consider later is effective. Equally effective and an essential component of the therapeutic process is supervision. Without appropriate and adequate supervision a therapist is not providing their best and most professional assistance to the client. It is the view of the authors that therapy without supervision is professionally unethical.

Another ethical issue is client representation or advocacy. As workers we endeavour to make informed choices and balanced decisions for and with our clients. Frequently, we become the decision maker as regards home care and support, and for placement in sheltered care. It is not so much the situations where we are the responsible agent for a client but the situations where we need to represent a client in a family dispute, which can present the most problematic issues for workers. Families can and do disagree on issues of care of their person with dementia. Due to their own distress in dealing with the dementia process, the irreversible changes in a loved one, family members may argue over what their parent requires in the way of care. We are the person with dementia's representative and as such we have a professional responsibility to ensure they have the best that can be provided for them in their situation and circumstances. The role of the worker could be as client advocate and family mediator. It is helpful at this point to consult with other service providers involved, to network wider, to ensure a holistic picture for management. Often peer group supervision and/or consultation is another valuable tool a worker can draw on and refer to.

Working with different ethnic groups

Another worker issue is representing the needs of the aged from different ethnic groups. For those who learnt a new language and culture, with the progress of dementia the frame of reference will not be the language and culture of their adopted country but that of their homeland. Despite popular myth it is no more possible for such a person to remain at home until death than it is for anyone else. Family support networks are usually far less extensive for migrant families than for those locally born. Extended family networks may have originally been able to provide the care for a person with dementia. Today the smaller nuclear family meeting the day-to-day demands of another culture is quite obviously less advantaged. This is particularly so as care provision in modern western culture is most often provided by a single person, usually a woman.

Cultural mores and religious beliefs and practices may further isolate carers and families. Support services that are sensitive to these needs are comparatively rare. The provision of these services need to be accessible if ethnic carers are to have a choice and avail themselves of a more equal share of community resources.

REFERENCES AND SUGGESTED READING

Carer, B. and McGoldrick, M. (1988) *The Changing Family Life Cycle* (2nd ed). New York: Gardner Press.

Compton, B. and Galway, B. (eds) (1979) *Social Work Processes*. Illinois: Peacock Publishers.

Gidley, I. and Shears, R. (1987) *Alzheimers*. Sidney: Allen and Unwin.

Goding, G. (1992) *The History and Principles of Family Therapy*. Melbourne: VAFT Publication.

Haley, J. (1976) *Problem Solving Therapy*. London: Harper Colophon.

Hoffman, L. (1981) *Foundations of Family Therapy*. New York: Basic Books.

McCallum, P. and Lang, M. (1989) *A Family Therapy*. Melbourne: Penguin Books.

McGoldrick, M. and Gerson, R. (1985) *Genograms in Family Assessment*. New York: Norton and Company.

Minuchin, S. (1974) *Families and Family Therapy*. London: Tavistock Publications.

The Networker (1988) Family Therapist Survey Results, Jan/Feb.

Pincus, A. and Minahan, A. (1973) *Social Work Practice: Model and Method*. Illinois: Peacock Publishers.

Turner, F. (1978) *Psychosocial Therapy*. London: Free Press.

POINTS FOR DISCUSSION

1. Is there in your experience a reluctance to apply systemic family intervention skills and methods to situations involving a person with dementia?

2. Discuss the frequency of the suggested indicators for situations where a systemic family intervention would be appropriate.

3. Consider situations known to you where the following might, or might not, be useful:
   - The Family Assessment Wheel
   - Contracts
   - Circular questioning
   - Genograms
   - Sculpting
   - Homework
   - Behaviour modification

4. How appropriate is client representation or advocacy in working with families where a member has dementia?

5. Discuss the point that 'cultural mores or religious beliefs and practices may further isolate carers and families'.

Chapter Five

Groupwork

Alan Chapman

INTRODUCTION

This chapter explores the influence of groups set up by professionals for a particular purpose. It will focus mainly on six support groups for carers of people with dementia. A seventh group which has adopted a self help approach is also considered since, unlike the others, it involves carers, people with dementia and volunteers and therefore provides a useful contrast to the professionally-led groups.

Networks of support are crucial for the carers of people with dementia. Support groups initiated by professionals have a part to play. However, an understanding of group processes, the needs of carers, and aims and purposes which are set out and reviewed regularly, require to be kept in mind by the new social worker. The message of this chapter is that support groups are no quick fix and cannot replace other more formal interventions.

What, then, is the purpose of groupwork with elderly people and in particular with carers of people with dementia? Two reasons given by social work and other professionals are the demands and pressures of caring for someone with dementia and the carer's increasing isolation from outside contact.

If a group can be defined as a 'plurality of individuals who are in contact with one another, who take one another into account and who are aware of some significant commonality' (Olmsted 1959) does this occur in practice? If a characteristic of the group is that it has 'open' membership this means that new members are recruited in a particular way. The open group is one which has a regular meeting time and invites anyone to come to the group, but recognises that the membership will change from meeting to meeting. As a result there may not be any long term commitment to the group by any one member.

Alternatively the 'closed' group may be one where the membership has, for instance, been restricted to those who have relatives with dementia as patients in a long stay hospital ward. The same individuals will attend each meeting, allowing more opportunity for the leader to work with them on an ongoing basis.

What type of leadership occurs? Is it directive and highly focused or non-directive and member-centred? Greening (quoted by Douglas 1986) suggests that leaders should initiate behaviour that positively demonstrates patterns of responses which will eventually move the group towards achieving its goals. Other researchers have tried to isolate the effects of leadership style on the interaction and satisfaction of group members. They found non-directive leaders to create more interaction within a group, and that the interaction was 'member-centred'. Non-directive leadership was characterised by the following:

- reflected the feelings of members
- gave support, praise or encouragement to members
- invited members to seek feedback
- summarised what had been said
- allowed group members to take responsibility for leading the group discussion

In contrast, directive leadership was defined by the following behaviours:

- the group was led verbally in discussion
- members were challenged and confronted
- members were exhorted
- suggested procedures were made for group members
- leaders evaluated or interpreted a response by a member

When considering support groups, the leaders (although initiating the meetings and setting the agenda) all had a common purpose to respond to the needs of the members. If new members have the important intimacy needs of being welcomed, valued, respected, listened to and encouraged to share feelings in a warm trusting environment, then predominantly the leadership style has to be non-directive.

In the primary group, members have warm, intimate and personal ties with one another, are usually small in number, face to face, spontaneous and devoted, although not necessarily explicitly, to mutual or common ends. The friendship group, and the family, are usually cited as foremost examples of primary groups. 'These groups then are the springs of life not only for the individual but for social institutions' Cooley (1909). Alternatively, the characteristics of the secondary group complement those of the primary group. Relations among members are cool, impersonal, rational, contractual and formal. Secondary groups are typically large and members have usually only intermittent contacts, often through the written rather than the spoken word. Examples range from the professional association to the large, bureaucratic corporation.

Common to all groups are the internal processes that occur as a result of the social interaction between individual group members. This is an area that is seldom given much attention by workers who bring people together with little thought about creating an appropriate climate for interaction. People come to groups with different expectations, needs and wants. Schutz (1959) suggests that inclusion, control and affection are the main interpersonal needs of a group member. The cohesiveness and process of control operating in a group can affect the wellbeing of the group members. For the new member the need for inclusion or feeling a sense of belonging to a group is influenced by the impact of the verbal and non-verbal behaviour of other members, particularly the leader and his or her behaviour within the group.

New group members watch the leader intently, as in an unfamiliar situation people tend to look for examples of acceptable and safe ways of behaving. The leader's function as a role model crucially affects what examples are used. If new members have the important intimacy needs of being welcomed, respected, valued, listened to and encouraged to share feelings in a warm, trusting environment then predominantly the leadership style has to be non-directive.

THE FAMILY AS CARERS

The family still plays a major role in meeting the needs of the elderly person. In a recent article George (1990) suggests that there are more than one and a quarter million people in the UK who care for disabled relatives. The dilemma for professionals is how to support the family network of care without unintentionally weakening their responsibilities. The majority of carers are women who, often at great cost to themselves, provide support and help for their relatives. This burden of caring is unremitting and is aptly described in *The Thirty Six Hour Day* (Mace 1985). The illness of dementia can create tensions in family relationships, particularly when a spouse sees their partner's personality and behaviour changing.

Typically, one person, usually the spouse, takes on the role of the main carer. As a result of the burden of caring they are often subject to a high degree of physical and psychological stress. It is therefore not unusual for carers to feel alone in their struggle with this progressive illness. Not only does the person with dementia begin to drift away from outside social contacts so, too, does the carer who needs to be constantly around. *The Thirty Six Hour Day* paints the picture: 'It may seem impossible to get out of the house, and life narrows down to a tight circle of lonely misery. Feelings of sadness and grief seem more painful when you feel alone with your problem'.

Similarly, the relative of someone with dementia may have to deal with what has been called the 'living bereavement' of coming to terms with the effects of dementia on the personality and functioning of the person they care for.

PRACTICAL HELP

It therefore becomes essential for the carer to find ways of caring for themselves that will allow a recharging of their emotional and physical resources. Professional groups such as British Association of Social Workers (BASW) and Social Care Association (SCA) and charities such as the Alzheimer's Disease Society/Alzheimers Scotland have recognised the importance of the support group as a way in which practical help can be given to carers. Gendron (1986) has hypothesised that the extent of the burden reported by carers is also a function of the effectiveness of the supporters' coping skills.

Various research studies have suggested that increased social support buffers the carers from the burdens of the care-giving role. Qualitative studies such as those done by Morris *et al.* (1989) have suggested that the efficacy of such networks has a complex interrelationship with the functioning of the carer.

Dunbar (1991) has indicated that from his analysis carer well-being is associated with the amount and quality of social support they experience. Carer groups are of importance as they provide some of this social support, often acting as a confidence booster as well as confirming ideas or offering suggestions about how they, as carers, should respond to their relative with dementia.

Social workers, like other professionals, have a vested interest in maintaining and utilising networks of support, since the essence of care management is that sensitive and appropriate interventions at the point where most needed involves utilising support networks. Consequently, one option, in addition to considering day centre attendance, residential home admissions and individual counselling, is often the support group. Whether initiated by a social worker, careworker or nurse, based in the community, residential home or day hospital, these groups have become a norm for practice.

A support group for family members can provide an opportunity for sharing experiences, and for help in resolving problems. To do so may help them understand and come to terms with the present level of functioning of the person with dementia. Through group discussion and meeting professionals the carer can begin to focus on ways of enhancing existing potential rather than dwelling on 'The person they once knew'.

As well as being faced with the task of caring, carers often face the problem of untangling and understanding the intricate and complex network of appropriate health or social services, and welfare benefits. Blockages are often experienced as carers try to get help.

GROUPS FOR PEOPLE WITH DEMENTIA

Much of the professionals' work with people with dementia in day centres, residential homes or long stay hospital wards is concerned with the management of their behaviour. As people who have different life experiences, likes and dislikes and personalities, the emphasis is placed on individual assessment and care plans, usually involving a key worker. This is done for the very good reason of trying to tailor the responses of staff to meet the needs of the resident whilst attempting to offset the institutionalising effect of being in a non-domestic setting.

The ability of staff to provide such an individualised service is dependent on staff numbers, teamwork and their motivation and morale. It is also likely that the manager of the unit or the staff themselves will engage in organised group activity as a means of both providing stimulation and coping with the demands of the residents.

Group activities are therefore seen as cost effective management in terms of staff time and the numbers of staff required. The bingo or domino session for the group of 20 residents or patients, overseen by two members of staff is often the norm for many settings. Such an approach denies some of the basics of groupwork. Although the elderly person may be a captive group member, should they not be consulted or have some choice in what they want to do? Undoubtedly, staff require skills of leadership so that they can enthuse and lead in a manner which takes account of what other individuals can offer. The elderly person with dementia who still has an ability to play the piano despite other communication difficulties often goes unnoticed by staff. Similarly, staff need to remind themselves that the resident or patient group has a 'life' of its own which can have a powerful effect on an individual's behaviour. For instance, why does one particular individual always sit in the one armchair or seem to be reluctant to do things for themselves?

All too often behaviour is attributed by staff to individualistic responses, personality traits, sheer awkwardness or attention seeking, with little attention given to the group influences. It is worth pausing to remember that for many residents or patients there was no real choice about where or with whom they would live and the reality is that they would not necessarily choose to associate with their fellow group member in the outside world. Burnside (1984) suggests that groupwork with elderly people involves a more directive approach on the part of the leader, partly because of their special problems, which must be recognised and dealt with.

Some older people have a preoccupation with loss and death: losses not only of their circle of friends but of physical abilities. Therefore a major objective in such groupwork is to alleviate this general anxiety by helping group members resolve these pre-occupations, rather than attempt to encourage new insights or personality changes. Such generalisations do not readily provide answers, particularly for those with dementia who may be disoriented of time and place, yet may know that they are not coping. Nevertheless, workers require to think seriously about their motivation and reasons for having groups.

Having established some baseline from which to evaluate the support groups, a description and analysis is given of the various groups.

THE SEVEN GROUPS

The seven groups used as part of the research for this chapter can be categorised in three main ways. Five of the groups can be termed professionally-led groups as they were initiated by professionals and involve carers. These groups are the Pines group, the long stay patient relative support group, the St. Margaret's carer and relative group, the Seaport group and the Riverside group. The sixth group, although initiated by a professional, adopted a 'therapeutic person-centred' approach and involved a trained Rogerian counsellor working with a small group of carers over a six week period. This group is called the Braeside group. The seventh group, unlike the others, is a self help group for people with dementia and their carers and does not involve any professionals.

Apart from the self-help group each was sent a short questionnaire (Appendix 8.1) and three of the leaders were interviewed. A short description of each group follows. The self-help group had been the subject of previous research by Foster (1991). This provided an extensive bank of information for this chapter.

The professionally-led support groups

The Pines group Hospital based, started in 1983 by the senior charge nurse of the day hospital for relatives of patients with dementia.

Main purpose: To allow a venue for relatives to discuss problems and give vent to feelings in a safe environment. This open group meets on a monthly basis, and involves the hospital social worker.

The long stay patient relative support group Hospital based, started in 1986 by the nursing staff and hospital social worker.

Main purpose: To continue to provide support to carers whose relatives had been admitted to the long stay ward. This open group meets monthly.

The St Margaret's carers' support group/relatives' support group Both groups are open and based in a residential home for people with dementia; started in 1990 and 1991 respectively, and led by the deputy officer, and officer in charge respectively. The carers' support group is for carers of relatives who are given respite care within the home. The relatives' support group is for those residents who are permanent in the home.

Main purpose (Both groups): Sharing and supporting one another and in response to carer distress.

The Riverside group A community based group set up in 1988 by interested professionals. Meets on a monthly basis in a non-institutional setting.

Main purpose: Support for carers, education and raising public awareness.

The Seaport group Set up in 1990 by a project worker from the social work department.

Main purpose: The purpose of the monthly association meetings were to find out local needs and what services carers wanted for their relative with dementia. A weekly Friday club is held for younger people with dementia and their carers. This group provides professional contact, friendship and support.

All of the groups had been initiated by professionals: a social worker, community psychiatric nurse, or day hospital nurse, and staff of a residential home. Similarly, all the group leaders stated that at least one of their aims was to provide an opportunity for friendship, education and problem solving.

Group membership

All the groups had begun with the carers of the person with dementia. For longer established groups, membership had been extended to other family members. To some extent, therefore, these support groups had restricted membership initially but could not be termed closed groups since those involved expressed the hope that other carers not in receipt of statutory services might hear about the group meetings. As an example, to further 'open' its meetings the Riverside group used the local media; they placed advertisements in the local newspaper, posters in health centres and GP surgeries and used the local radio station to promote the formation of itself in the community. Professionals are extensively involved as leaders and are part of the local Alzheimers' branch.

Group purpose

The most commonly stated reason for initiating a support group was the recognition that carers often felt distressed and isolated as a result of caring for a relative with dementia. This psychological distress is reported by carers as being a result of not knowing what to expect, inadequate information about dementia or feeling unsure in how to deal with particular behaviour. Consequently, the support group had some notion of educating carers by increasing their knowledge and awareness. Significantly, this seemed not to extend to creating self-sufficient groups independent of staff. However, a second benefit perceived by professional staff was that relatives could provide mutual support to one another, by sharing experiences but also having a safe environment in which to give vent to feelings of frustration and guilt, with people who understood.

This is not dissimilar to Toseland's (1990) view that time needs to be spent with carers dealing with their emotions and feelings, their reaction to their relative with dementia and their need for self-care to avoid 'burn-out'.

Burnside (1984) states similar reasons but adds that to educate the family about the pathological processes occurring in the person with dementia can help them to realign their expectations of their relative and so focus on existing potential. Clearly, with carers the goals of the group will be determined by their particular experience with the person who has dementia. As the members become acquainted with each other, opportunities will arise to gain mutual support from peers but also enhanced self-esteem. Burnside suggests that this can enable a sense of intimacy and trust to develop as members assuage guilt, alleviate feeling of grief and share in accomplishments of coping with behaviour. Although leaders indicated that carers derived benefits from attending group meetings, I gained the distinct impression that scant attention is paid to the forming stage of groups when purposes, commitment and trust are agreed by all present.

The Pines group serves as an example. In this group the phenomenon of the graduate carer evolved. These carers had attended the group for a long time but their relative had died or moved on to another setting. They were invited by the leaders to continue to attend the group meetings as part of their continuing support, although group membership was restricted to relatives of patients with dementia attending the day hospital. Unfortunately, it quickly became apparent that a mismatch existed in the group purposes. Whilst the ideal model conceived by the leaders was one where the graduate carers would help new highly stressed carers to work through their feelings about their relative having dementia, in reality the graduate carers did not want to be reminded of a traumatic and painful past. They therefore saw the group as an extension of their network of leisure and social activity.

A disadvantage of this group then became that of the new versus the old, with the latter using the group for purposes other than those intended by the leaders. This seems to confirm the view that a group essentially reforms every time it meets because of the intervening life events for each of its members. Had the leaders at an early stage of the group taken account of these changing needs, perhaps the situation in which new members found that they had nothing in common with existing members could have been avoided.

Similarly, the expectations, and pressures arising from the many 'ups' and 'downs' of caring for a loved one moving through the various stages of dementia and associated behavioural changes, leads to a changed group from meeting to meeting. Most of the carer groups met monthly and, although not specifically researched, the impression gained was that the leaders followed their planned programmes rather than considering the developing life of the group. The leadership of the group then becomes a crucial factor.

Group leadership

In all cases the leaders of the group remained the professionals. This is understandable, since they initiated most groups. This means that the professional, as often as not, orchestrates the meetings in a fairly directive way, perhaps involving the carers in particular tasks. The dilemma then becomes at what point do leaders become non directive and 'let go' and allow the members scope to develop in their particular ways. Of course the risk attached to letting go is that the group will cease to meet, thus adding extra pressures on workers as they are faced with providing one-to-one support, education and information. If the creation of dependency by members on the leaders was consciously tackled in the early stages of the group, members could be enabled to view the group as a shared responsibility with an evolving and increasing role for carer control.

Group activities

The meetings of most groups were held monthly throughout the year, with social activities at festive and other occasions. The Riverside group, however, had also embarked on 'political' activity by becoming a community care watchdog intent on asserting the needs of people with dementia and their carers with local service providers. An example of a support group meeting is as follows:

Introduction to group

Speaker – for example doctor, pharmacist, community worker.
(In one group the speaker is encouraged to enter into discussions after a short presentation).

Informal discussion over cup of coffee/tea.

Recap the main points of the meeting.

Adjourn to bar for further 30–45 minutes for the professionals to engage in 1:1 'problem solving' with individuals. Carers could then socialise on a more informal basis.

For the group based in a day hospital the intention was to allow carers the opportunity to meet senior medical staff so that they could put faces to names, whilst learning about dementia.

Perceived benefits
Implicit in all support groups seemed to be the notion of honesty on the part of professionals in letting carers know the failing situation of the people with dementia, so that the group could then begin to help them cope. Consequently, one worker talked of the 'pressure cooker' function, in that carers could 'let off steam' with people who shared a common experience. The awareness raising aspect of groups was seen as important so that carers might have accurate information. Finally, carers were seen as having enhanced self-esteem because they were listened to, valued as individuals, taken seriously and encouraged to share difficulties without feeling a sense of failure and guilt.

The self-help group
To offer some comparison with the professionally-led groups, attention will now be given to the self-help group which operates a weekly drop-in club for people with dementia and their carers and is staffed by volunteers.

The club first met in 1989 and was initiated by a married couple who had recent experience of looking after an elderly relative with dementia and had been involved in the setting up of a local Alzheimer's branch. Frustrated by the lack of progress on getting funds for a more formal project, and seeing the demand for day care for people with early onset dementia and their carers, the weekly drop-in club was established. The most notable feature of the club's development is that it was almost entirely achieved on a voluntary basis by people who were not professionally employed or qualified to do such work. This has influenced the character of the club which is run on the principle that nobody is in charge and all members have an equal say in what is done. Though not titled a support group, and although members might deny that groupwork takes place, some of the functions have a similarity to support groups. For instance, there is practical help in terms of advice on medication, behavioural problems, local contacts and resources.

This is not dissimilar to the views of Katz and Levin (1980) about the growth of the self help movement. They suggest that this has occurred because of a depersonalisation and over-specialisation of services which has led to a general loss of confidence in their ability to provide comprehensive care. Unlike the professionally-led groups, every group member is in some degree a leader. Certainly the organisers, who are the driving force behind the group, appear to take no real leadership role, other than organising the venue. So what attracts the users to the club?

Group membership

No statutory service existed for carers of people with early onset dementia. Those with dementia and their carers attend the club together. Users initially came from the carers' support group run by the Alzheimer's branch, who retain overall control of the club. Membership criteria is dependent on the person with dementia being diagnosed as having dementia. The club does not restrict its membership to people with a marked degree of dependency but regards itself as existing for people of all ages who have dementia. Carers tend to find out about the club by word of mouth from the branch or current group members.

Limits to the membership are imposed by the maximum of ten people permitted to use the community lounge in a sheltered housing complex.

The aims of the club were given as follows:

1. To allow carers to continue to socialise in a context where they feel at ease with sufferers.

2. To combat the isolation that many carers feel.

3. To provide socialisation for the carer and sufferer.

Because of the small numbers, the activities are in response to members' suggestions. Carers are not expected to do any of the work involved: the idea being to give them a break, and it is intended to provide an environment where people need not be embarrassed by the way people with dementia behave.

Group activities

These were identified in terms of: (1) practical needs, (2) social and emotional needs, and (3) educational needs. The main activity is talking, exchanging news about the past week and suggestions about problems may be raised. Whilst much of the talk is about Branch activities and the problems that dementia brings, people at the club have a strong interest in each other's lives and interests. Mutual support is possible as carers tell each other about the information they have gained about resources, services and so forth.

Although similar to the professional-led support group this informal approach filled a gap in services for people with early onset dementia. The coming together weekly for a sit-down meal is an important focus of the day.

Perceived benefits

Members interviewed indicated that the club met its own aims by providing a social occasion for both carers and people with dementia which combated the isolation that they may otherwise have experienced. Members talked of the club as something they enjoyed and in which they were able to relax with others whom they knew well. The club was also a place where carers could go as a couple and the behaviour of the relative with dementia was understood and accepted. People at the club treated each other in an ordinary and respectful way. Especially for carers, this compensated for the misunderstandings, loneliness and pain they experienced elsewhere. Consequently, they were able to give vent to the frustrations of caring with other group members.

A problem-solving process also took place, usually around the sharing of a particular situation. This presented dilemmas for some members concerning the right of the carer to talk about the person with dementia in front of them. Their concern was that the person with dementia might pick up on general conversation and become distressed and angered by being talked about.

The advantages of the club is that it can be flexible and responsive to the needs of its users without the delay imposed by a bureaucratic and hierarchical structure. This raises the disadvantage that volunteers may find it hard to sustain a high level of involvement, especially when un-met needs are discovered. Resources are limited and expertise is needed. This may place unreasonable demands on volunteers who may find it difficult to establish boundaries for their roles. The club has to ration places and this means that people who might benefit are unable to attend.

There is little doubt that the drop-in club makes a valuable contribution to users' lives because it exemplifies an approach where people with dementia and their carers are valued as individuals with varied human needs. However, a question remains as to whether the carers' needs for support complement the interests of people with dementia or not. Nevertheless, I do not advocate that new social workers sit back and have nothing to do with carers' support groups! One lesson from the self-help example is that carers have a lot to offer and should be encouraged to utilise experience in helping others in practical, emotional and social ways. The new social worker requires to work in partnership and collaboratively rather than feel they must always initiate and control.

The Braeside group

The final group that will be considered is the Braeside group. Unlike the other groups this was initiated by the manager of a resource centre for people with dementia, as a response to requests from carers. Significantly, the expressed purpose was to assist carers be independent of staff and to make use of their own abilities and knowledge.

The Braeside group was set up in 1990 by the then officer in charge: The group was educative but arose from a desire to respond to relatives' needs for a more 'Therapeutic, person-centred service'. The objective was not to have relatives solely dependent on the staff of this resource centre for people with dementia.

The manager of the resource unit for people with dementia was concerned about those people who did not want to join a carers' support group of 20–26 people. There were also some carers expressing a wish for a more therapeutic person-centred service. An experienced Rogerian counsellor was involved with the manager in leading sessions for a group of five or six carers on a two weekly basis over a six month period.

The Rogerian approach assumes that individuals have the innate potential to resolve and learn to deal with their own problems on an emotional level. The purposes of this group were to provide a forum which gave carers an opportunity to discuss the varied emotions caused by coping with the person with dementia. It was the intention that the group would recognise that circumstances and problems were different for each member and that meant that each would have to find an individual way of coping. The membership of the group was drawn from the larger support group with numbers limited to six over a six month period. These same six members attended every meeting and therefore formed a closed group.

As the group progressed, the members felt safe in beginning to discuss the limits of their personal tolerance, patience and awareness concerning decisions about care for their relative. Feelings of anger, frustration and rejection as well as sadness were expressed as group members were encouraged to look objectively at their situation.

The professional counsellor along with the officer in charge remained the leaders of the group. They adopted the role of facilitators, encouraging an open expression of feelings. From an intensive therapeutic approach the members moved on to begin a fund raising committee for social activities at the centre as well as attending educational training.

Perceived benefits?
The group members formed strong bonds, and started to meet each other outside group sessions. They established shared interests and activities which enabled them to be less constrained by their carer role. This meant that they were not dependent on the resource centre staff to help them deal with crisis issues.

Significantly, these group members were regarded as having the inner resources to cope with their personal emotional problems as a result of the sessions and, unlike the main support group, became much less reliant on the professional staff.

Having completed a critique of the seven groups there are a number of issues central to the running of support groups which now need to be identified. These issues represent my view of what the new social worker needs to bear in mind when thinking about setting up a support group.

SUMMARISING THE CENTRAL ISSUES

This chapter begun by raising some questions about support groups. These questions related to whether attending a group for a carer enhances their support networks and, perhaps more fundamentally, actually addresses their personal needs and the requirements arising from their caring circumstances.

The professionals' understanding of group processes and the need for clarity about group purposes were highlighted as crucial aspects of a support group's effectiveness. So what have we learned?

Any group that is organised, in my view exists for the realisation of the purposes and goals of its members, and these will vary from group to group and from time to time within a single group. The group, therefore, is simply the means by which members are enhanced through the achievement of their stated purposes.

We have focused on three main approaches to providing group support for carers of people with dementia. If a group is to be effective, as can be seen from all the examples, a clear sense of purpose is important. This purpose should reflect the wishes of all participants as well as reflect the concerns that they have as carers. However, any group, as it meets, begins to evolve in terms of the relationships between the members. Although members differ widely in their ability to influence the group, new leaders can emerge. People with particular knowledge, experience, or interpersonal skills have an important role in sustaining the group and need to be given encouragement. So for the new social worker there is a need to understand that groups are living 'energy' systems and that, once initiated, groups can develop in ways unforeseen by the leader.

Learning about group interaction requires a basic understanding of the 'network of intertwining systems of events of memories, of experience, of current perceptions which underlay the simplest of situations' (Douglas 1986).

In terms of the support groups considered, distinct models exist, but the common objective is to alleviate stress in carers. There is no doubt that although support groups are important for carers, conflicts are inevitable, particularly when there are differences of interests, desires, goals or values. Consequently, the exercise of power and status by the professional can either lead to the group being dependent or, alternatively, work towards being self-sustaining. Perhaps one lesson from this chapter is that the group which enabled carers to retain their own individual solutions was the Braeside group which intensively focused on feelings and encouraged a personal response to other group members and their situations. The professionals acted as enablers so that the 'group members formed strong bonds and started to meet on other occasions than the group sessions'. Although you may question the validity of the participants becoming a fund-raising group, the important point to emphasise is that this is what they wanted to do.

Predominantly, the support groups were professionally led, and yet they filled an important role in the networks of support for carers of people with dementia. Nevertheless, support groups cannot be a substitute for the provision of services, neither should the new social worker think that initiating a group replaces the more formal counselling and individual support that some carers will require. Support groups play a part, but demand time, planning, a serious consideration of purposes and an understanding of the leadership role.

However, it is worth noting that the self-help group was set up in response to a lack of leadership by professionals. Undoubtedly, the weekly meeting of this group, which allows the person with dementia and their carer to attend together, is an important support. The apparent strength of this group is that carers can help each other compensate for the misunderstanding, loneliness and pain they experienced elsewhere. It seems to me that the dilemma for the social worker is whether such carers gain the correct information, and understand the complexity of the reasons for behaviour of someone with dementia and are helped to cope.

Many new workers may feel uneasy at not knowing what is happening in such a group, particularly if they perceive a carer to be requiring support. I suspect the temptation is for workers to take over or usurp the existing leadership. This may be inappropriate but it has to be recognised that there is no single or right approach to providing help to carers. Any strategy is dependent on finding out what carers need from talking with carers.

As has been shown, caring for someone with dementia is a relentless burden for the carer which often leads to social isolation and withdrawal from everyday life, particularly for the spouse of someone with dementia. The emotional stresses and strains of such caring are well acknowledged, and it is in such a situation that a support group can become a welcome release for a carer to share with others. Intimacy and trust has to evolve through careful and sensitive leadership on the part of professionals.

CONCLUSIONS

Networks of support are important for the carer of people with dementia. Support groups, initiated by professionals, have a part to play. However, an understanding of the needs of carers and group processes are required and need to be considered and reviewed regularly by the worker. It has to be recognised that support groups, regardless of who acts as prime mover, are only a small part of the carers' everyday life.

The challenge for the new social worker is to create support groups which are not an end in themselves, but help the carer utilise the various networks of the wider community and so assist them in their caring task.

REFERENCES

Burnside, I. (1984) *Working with the Elderly: Group Process and Techniques, 2nd edition*. California: Wadsworth Health Sciences Division.

Cooley, C.H. (1909) *Social Organisation*. New York: Scribner and Sons.

Douglas, T. (1986) *Group Living*. London: Tavistock Publications.

Dunbar, M. (1991) Correlates of the well being of dementia care givers: A Meta-analysis (paper) presented at *B P S Health, Psychology Conference*. Nottingham University.

Foster, K. (1991) *The Kilmarnock Drop-In Centre*. Stirling: Dementia Services Development Centre.

Gendron, C.E. (1986) Skills training with supporters of the demented. *Journal of American Geriatrics Society* 34: 875–880.

George, A., Jackson, M. and George, J. (1990) The Never Ending Day-Community Outlook.

Katz, A. and Levin, E. (1980) Self care is not a solipsistic trap: A reply to critics. *International Journal of Health Services* 10(2) 329–336.

Mace, N.L., Rabins, P.V., Castleton, B.A., Cloke, C. and McEwen, E. (1985) *The Thirty Six Hour Day*. London: Age Concern.

Morris, R.G., Morris, L.W. and Britton, P.G. (1989) Factors affecting the emotional well-being of caregivers of dementia. *British Journal of Psychiatry* 153, 147–156.

Olmsted, M. (1959) *The Small Group*. New York: Random House.

Schutz, W.C. (1959) *F.I.R.O.* New York: Holt, Rinehart and Winston.

Toseland, R. (1990) Long term effectiveness of peer-led and professional-led support groups to care givers. *Social Service Reviews*. Chicago: University of Chicago.

Titmuss, R.M. (ed) (1958) *Essays on the Welfare State*. London: Allen and Unwin.

POINTS FOR DISCUSSION

1. What are the relative advantages and disadvantages of open and closed groups for supporting (i) carers of people with dementia? (ii) people with dementia?

2. Can the professional member of a support group he has initiated let go of the leadership role?

3. What are the most important points to emerge from the comparisons between the professional-led groups cited?

4. Discuss the proposition that learning about group interaction requires a basic understanding of the 'network of intertwining systems of events, of memories, of experience, of current perceptions which underlay the simplest of situations' (Douglas 1968).

CHAPTER SIX

Issues Arising from Two Contrasting Life Styles

Katrina Myers and Philip Seed

In this chapter we compare the lives of two elderly people with dementia living in very different circumstances. Mrs Smith lives in a residential home, her husband having recently given up the task of trying to care for her in their own house. Mrs Jones left a flat to live with her daughter and is able to manage, thanks to the daughter's ability and willingness to continue to support her. Both Mrs Smith and Mrs Jones are in their eighties and both could be described as suffering from moderate to severe dementia. Both are also in contact with other members of their families.

The lives of these two people are studied with particular reference to their social networks. These are produced using evidence from interviews and from daily diaries kept for fortnightly periods.

Mrs Smith

Mrs Smith, aged eighty, lived with her husband until recently being admitted to a residential home. The main difficulties at their own home had reflected Mrs Smith's deteriorating condition: a combination of wandering, inability to distinguish day and night, poor concentration and dressing difficulties. Mr Smith had been supported by members of a carers' group and by Crossroads. He had had periods of relief when Mrs Smith had received residential respite. It was his continued lack of sleep that led immediately to the decision that Mrs Smith should be admitted to a home on a long term basis.

Mr Smith, however, had some difficulty letting his wife leave him. He still feels responsible for his wife's behaviour.

Mrs Smith can still do some things for herself. She can eat independently, but her small concentration span makes more complex tasks difficult and she becomes impatient with herself. Within the home she has a bed-sit and to a certain extent she can keep it tidy, but not consistently so. Her reading and writing abilities are now very limited. She can no longer manage public transport without support and she cannot manage money.

Figure 6.1 shows the overall boundaries of Mrs Smith's social network. Within the home she meets staff, other residents and visitors. Her only visits out are to her husband and local walks with staff and other family visitors.

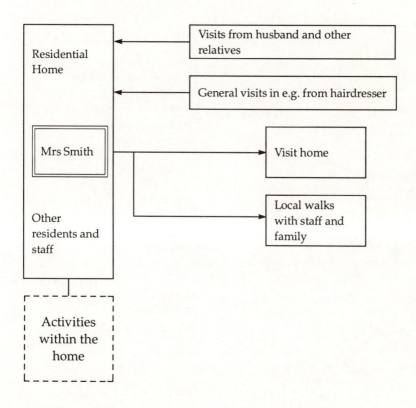

Figure 6.1: The overall boundaries of Mrs Smith's social network

Figure 6.2 gives a more detailed picture, dividing Mrs Smith's activities into personal activities (self-care) and social activities. It may be noted that the hairdresser visits the home rather than Mrs Smith going out to the hairdresser in the community. Her visitors include a number of different relatives while her social activities within the home are extensive with an emphasis on social mixing with her peer group. For example, there are some games with one or more individuals and some larger group activities such as a sing-song. This must be a very different life from her earlier life at home with her husband.

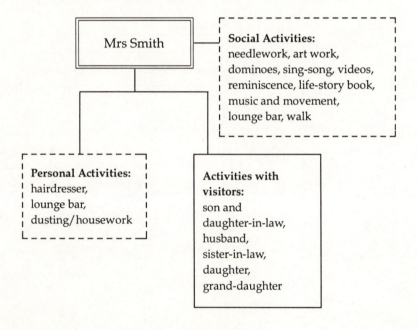

Figure 6.2: Mrs Smith's activities at the home

Figure 6.3 looks at Mrs Smith's significant social contacts in more detail. In spite of the number of relatives and the continuing contact with her husband, significant contacts within the home with staff and fellow residents are about twice as numerous. The number of different care staff to whom she relates helps to account for the large range of different kinds of social activities she engages in, shown in Figure 6.2, since different staff bring their own interests to the relationships. The relatives state that Mrs Smith's lifestyle has widened since she came to the home, giving her more freedom within a safe environment.

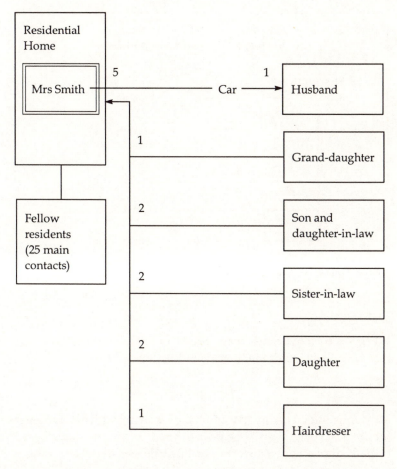

Figure 6.3: Mrs Smith's significant social contacts (based on diaries for two weeks).

On the other hand, as Figure 6.4 shows, the geographical space within which these contacts are made is very limited. Mrs Smith travels from her bedsit to a communal lounge and to a conservatory. Occasionally she walks within the immediate locality. The longest distance travelled is to her own old home and this only occurred once during the fortnight for which diaries were kept.

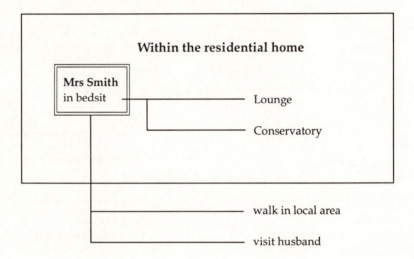

Figure 6.4: Spatial boundaries of Mrs Smith's social world

We will return to discuss these points, but first let us compare Mrs Smith's lifestyle with the lifestyle of Mrs Jones.

Mrs Jones

Mrs Jones is aged eighty five and has been living with her daughter for the past year. Figure 6.5 shows her pattern of daily living based on daily diaries kept for a fortnight. It will be seen that she continues to participate in daily domestic activities but her daughter says she has problems; for example forgetting things, not knowing where she is going, having to be checked and, in particular, not being able to make decisions for herself. Mrs Jones is often awake during the night and has to be checked, for example, in case she should set fire to something. In short her daughter has to support her at home in many ways and accompany her out of doors.

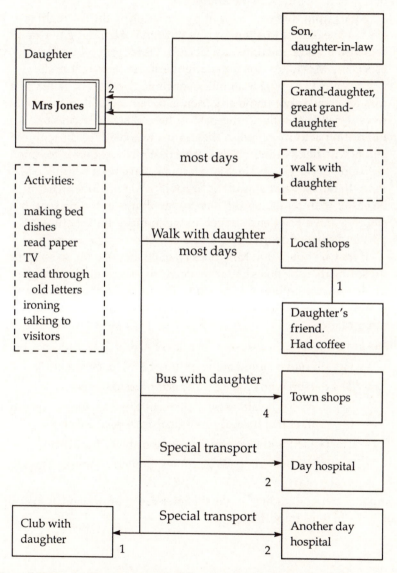

Figure 6.5: Mrs Jone's pattern of daily living (based on diaries kept for a fortnight)

Mrs Jones's life follows a weekly routine. This includes visits most days to the local shops, twice weekly visits to town shops by bus and weekly visits to two separate day hospitals. Transport is provided for the last named so that the daughter gets some respite during these periods, from 9.30am to 3.30pm or longer, in the case of one of the centres, in the afternoon.

Apart from this very regular pattern, during the fortnight covered by the diaries Mrs Jones visited a friend of her daughter's and was also accompanied to a social club. Visits from other relations, especially Mrs Jones' son and daughter-in-law also featured.

So far as her own social life is concerned, it may be noted that Mrs Jones does not name any friends of her own other than relatives. Friends belong to the past rather than to the present. An interesting activity noted in the diaries was reading through old letters with her daughter. Thinking of past relationships is common with elderly people and in this case it may have been helpful to Mrs Jones to refresh, and stimulate, her ability to remember. That may be easier than remembering day-to-day things in the present, but she may have been encouraged to try to make links between the past and current people, places and activities.

It may be noted that Mrs Jones is totally dependent on support for seeing that she takes her drugs correctly, to prompt her memory in day-to-day living; for example for food, clothes, managing money and, as we have stressed, taking decisions about these and other matters.

This example illustrates the essential roles of a carer of Mrs Jones at home:

- Her pivotal position at the centre of Mrs Jones' network
- The person who enables other activities to happen
- The person who alone can help to sustain Mrs Jones's quality of life in all of its physical, emotional and social aspects
- The person with a continuing responsibility for Mrs Jones
- A relative providing (as daughter) limited connections with the past

Compared to her daughter's role, the roles of the professionals are minimal, but still very important:

- Visits from the GP
- Attendance at day centres, giving both stimulation and a change of scene for Mrs Jones and respite for her daughter

There can sometimes be problems in the close relationship with her daughter. In the past Mrs Jones was 'meticulous' over small things and can become angry if things like clothes are not laid out as they should be. But in general there is mutual respect and affection and Mrs Jones often praises her daughter.

Amongst the issues this example immediately raises are the following:

1. Mrs Jones is very dependent on a single carer. Could the load be spread any more to enable the daughter to lead more of her own independent life?

2. Could there be more variety in the kinds of contacts Mrs Jones has? A problem may be that her contemporaries are likely to be physically frail and not so mobile.

3. In the light of the above, is access to suitable transport a problem for Mrs Jones? She is able to use the local bus to go accompanied by her daughter to the town shops, but that seems to be the limit of visits beyond a short walking distance, apart from special transport provided for hospital visits.

4. Mrs Jones is able to walk short distances with someone to accompany her and this seems to be a strength to be used for as long as possible. Walking, indeed, and visiting shops are really her only remaining informal outside interests.

5. Do we need to give further attention to the daughter's needs? If so, what forms of respite or additional support would help? Is a carers' group where the daughter could meet others in similar circumstances available?

A COMPARISON BETWEEN THE SOCIAL NETWORKS OF MRS SMITH IN A RESIDENTIAL SETTING AND MRS JONES AT HOME

Mrs Smith's network is almost an inverse of Mrs Jones's. By this we mean that Mrs Smith's is rich within her own home living environment and sparse outside. The opposite is true for Mrs Jones. She does little at home, has few visitors, but does many more things outside her home. These contrasts are shown in Figure 6.6:

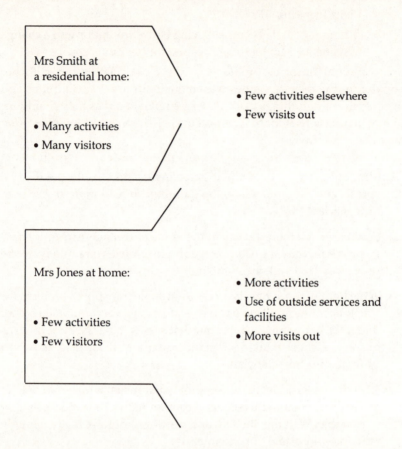

Figure 6.6: Contrasts between main locations of social contacts and activities for Mrs Smith and for Mrs Jones

Are these contrasts inevitable features of living in a residential setting and living with a relative at home? For example, does the hairdresser *have* to visit the residents rather than their visiting the hairdresser? Does it *have* to be the accepted norm that people tend to visit their relatives in residential establishments when they might be enabled to invite them into their own homes in the community? Approaching such questions from a quality of life perspective, we can suggest the need for opportunities both at home and outside, as shown in Figure 6.7:

At home	Outside
• Many opportunities	Many opportunities
• Many visitors	Variety of visits
• Range of activities	Range of activities

Figure 6.7: Maximum opportunities for enhancing quality of life

The difficulties in the way of developing Mrs Smith' activities outside the home are in terms of demands on staff time, as well as, perhaps, in traditional attitudes. (This is not to suggest that all residents should be 'forced' to go out more, even if staff were available.)

On the other hand, we may ask questions about Mrs Jones's outside activities. Were opportunities missed for developing friendships in the local community on account of the fact that both of the day centres she attended were hospital rather than community-based?

In short, one wants to know, can one have the best of both kinds of situation, whether the client lives at home, thanks to the support potential of a relative, or in a residential establishment, being able to incorporate some of the benefits otherwise associated with living at home? And can the undoubted social enrichment of living in a lively and simulating residential establishment be incorporated within a home-based network? These are the challenges raised by these two examples.

CHAPTER SEVEN

Empowerment

Alan Chapman

Although there is not much social work literature about empowerment the word is intuitively appealing; it sounds 'right'. It somehow reflects altruistic notions of consumer power, advocacy; or of the powerless and vulnerable becoming less so in an increasingly market economy approach to the provision of health and social services. Empowering people is also equated with providing the financial means so that they can exercise choice in the market place. Of course having choice is dependent on knowing that other alternative options exist.

A dictionary definition of empowerment suggests it means 'giving power or authority to, giving ability to, enabling, permitting'. Latin *potere* means 'to be able'. So in a broad sense empowerment is a process whereby people, organisations and communities gain mastery over their own social situations. In this chapter empowerment is taken to be a concept that embraces notions of individual rights, advocacy, power, and relates to our experience of life and being in charge of situations we find ourselves.

Empowerment is rooted in the idea of self-help or social action perspectives and implies that many competencies are present or possible given niches or windows of opportunity. This is not a real life picture since, though we may as individuals have demands for empowerment, it is nurtured by the effects of collaborative efforts. Kieffer (1984) suggests that it is a long term process of ordered and progressive development of participatory skills and political understanding that parallels our development from infancy through to adulthood.

In other words, as an infant our participation in the world is exploratory, dealing with the unknown, whilst the authority and power structures are demystified as a result of our explorations. The infant who purposely upturns the cup of milk onto the carpet is likely quickly to recognise that their parents are displeased and can exert authority over his/her freedoms! In the adult stage we integrate new personal knowledge and skills into the reality of our everyday life world. We develop a critical awareness of the root causes of problems and a readiness to act on our awareness. So, as an example, we become concerned by the threat to the ozone layer and react by joining in pressure group action, join the Green Party or switch to public transport instead of using our car!

Empowerment is not easy, given the many complex situations that workers have to deal with. For example,the patient with dementia who has been in a long stay hospital ward for a number of years will undoubtedly have an entirely different view and response to the idea of moving to live in the community, compared with the person who already lives in their own home. Although he or she may feel inappropriately placed in hospital, they may lack individual power to assert their view and may be subject to staff attitudes and prejudices because of being labelled a 'dementia patient'. It is more than likely in the hospital situation that decisions are made by those who have political, financial or professional power and therefore their interests may not coincide with those of the patient.

Whatever method or social work theory the social worker uses, he or she essentially intervenes in the life situation of a client to bring about some change in the client's position. A standard description of the social work task could read 'Good or effective, social work is not simply "doing things" for the client, it is more "doing things alongside" the client – working with the client in co-operation to bring about positive change' (Tossell and Webb 1986). This task, the helping relationship, although apparently simple, is complex because it is difficult for one person to know what is for the 'good' of another. So conflicts of interest exist between the worker and the client. People who are in vulnerable situations and need help may be bitter and resentful of the fact that they cannot cope. They may want things to change yet at times may want to keep things as they are.

EMPOWERMENT AND THE SOCIAL WORKER'S ROLE
Essentially the role of the worker is to deal with managing situations of tension, of uncertainty, dependency, impossibility, and differences of interest which have elements of '...living with and surviving...but also

of doing something about' (Clough 1990). This has been termed case advocacy where the social worker gives 'privacy to the interests of individual clients' (Turner 1977).

Staff who view themselves as an advocate face an unwritten tension. They work for social service departments, and are not employed directly by service users. Therefore the objectives of the department for particular client groups may not necessarily coincide with the requirements of service users. Workers then face making judgements about the interests of different parties, be it the person with dementia or their carer. Consequently, workers are not able to achieve what they would like because, as Clough (1990) indicates, 'personal social services cannot rectify intractable problems... which arise from the fact that some people have worse life opportunities in terms of income, housing; education and health'.

Nevertheless, such a scenario has not stopped workers devising ways of attempting to bridge the gulf between the client and themselves. We will focus on the task-centred casework approach because it attempts to tackle problems experienced by clients by means of a contract and the setting of specific achievable tasks. One of the perceived strengths of this approach is that it concentrates on the user's own conception of his or her difficulties as this holds the key to reaching a solution. At first glance it might be assumed that the user was being empowered. However, the reality of the social casework approach is that the worker usually identifies the users' deficits in functioning and development. The task-centred approach then enters into a contract with the person which implicitly empowers.

However, the reaching of an acceptable solution poses the question in who defines 'acceptable' – the worker or the individual? As Perlman (1957) states 'The goal of case work is... to help people achieve socially constructive and individually satisfying lives'.

APPLICATION TO WORK WITH PEOPLE WITH DEMENTIA

People with dementia are an example of users who, because of their illness, are stigmatised and subject to others taking control over their life. This has been referred to as the disabling relationship, where the person with dementia is made to be dependent on others. The label of dementia for carers and social workers conjures up the picture of someone who is unable to function or cope with everyday living tasks. Although this may be so in the later stages of having dementia, in the earlier stage the person may have retained skills and abilities despite losses in other areas of their functioning. Empowerment of the person with dementia is problematic, yet the worker has to be careful not to fall into the trap of thinking it does not matter.

Although the process of being empowered entails interactions with others which strengthen and benefit our personal networks within society, it also inherently has the notion of power status and degree of economic wealth. The care in the community legislation (NHS and Community Care Act 1990) is based on the premise that users of services should have power shared with them.

A MONOPOLY OF RESPONSIBILITY?

The social worker must be aware of the power they possess, based on knowledge and learning, particularly when intruding into people's personal lives. The new worker should examine ways that can release some of their power to help those who may be vulnerable, lack status in society and have little wealth. Interventions to empower, therefore, must take account of the other factors which influence an individual's ability to deal with a particular problem. The social worker does not have a monopoly of responsibility for resolving a particular situation as other networks of support and other professionals can be utilised by the user. For empowering individuals the following points can be noted.

1. Individuals need to be respected in that they have the capacity and ability to make decisions, act on their own behalf, and often know what changes have to be made to allow them to direct their own destinies. People can empower themselves!

2. Social workers may need to surrender their need for control and link in with networks of support in a co-operative and collaborative manner.

3. There is a need for mutual respect and a recognition by the worker that the client may reject the help that is offered. The relationship is not one sided.

4. If empowerment is to be a collaborative process then imbalances of power must be exposed as they prohibit people from achieving their full potential.

5. Social workers should secure and use resources that will promote or foster a sense of control and promote individual ability.

   6. Adopt a person-valuing approach, building in the important
      condition of trust.

If workers are to subscribe to an empowerment model then they need to
legitimise the beliefs that people are equal partners in the network of care.
This requires a reframing of thinking about the role and moving from
being only a provider of service and controller of resources to becoming
a facilitator, enabler and resource for clients to use. It is the results of self
awareness, self growth and access to resources that empower the client –
not the services provided. The Care in the Community legislation (Community Care Act 1990) embraces such notions, although the individual
development of users is implicit rather than explicitly stated.

ADOPTING AN EMPOWERING APPROACH – A CASE EXAMPLE

Aunt Emily had come to stay ten years previously, uninvited, after the
death of her sister. Mr and Mrs Allen were her only relatives. At first there
were no problems but gradually Emily began to be forgetful, took to
getting up in the middle of the night to do housework and washing,
became disoriented and incontinent. This culminated in her leaving gas
taps on the cooker turned on but not lit, continually soiling her clothes
and neglecting her own personal hygiene. Mrs Allen stormed out of the
house one day saying she could take no more and something required to
be done.

   Workers, when faced with this situation and the question 'what do you
do?' in training sessions usually talk about doing an assessment. Whilst
this may indeed be a correct response, there exists a tension between what
the two main actors in this situation require. Emily may need some
involvement from a medical practitioner, in order to determine what
might be treatable. Mrs Allen needs something different. This might be
counselling, information about dementia, and practical support.

   It may be inappropriate for Emily to be immediately removed to a
residential home/nursing home which would create disruption in her
routines and life and leave Mrs Allen feeling she has failed in some way.
Adopting an empowering approach might mean that the worker shares
various options and choices with both Mrs Allen and Emily. The worker
might usefully discover what they saw the difficulty as being and they
may find possible solutions, using the supports available in the situation.
Although such a scenario is hypothetical, the point of the exercise is to

have workers explore courses of action in which the consumers are being listened to and helped to retain control over their circumstances.

Consequently, it may become apparent that social networks and support systems need to be strengthened so that self-care efforts are enhanced rather than impeded and made more burdensome. Similarly, social workers, by virtue of their expertise and knowledge, are in powerful positions. Rather than impose their expertise on clients, this knowledge can be used as a tool for empowerment. Undoubtedly a certain amount of risk taking is involved, but social workers need to remember that often the person with dementia and/or their carer knows what's best and knows the most about the changes they have to make.

EMPOWERMENT FOR THE PERSON WITH DEMENTIA

For the person with dementia, the manifestation of their illness causes those around them to take an ever increasing control over decisions, daily living tasks and communication. Carers and social workers respond to the increasing deficits and difficulties they observe the person with dementia facing. People get caught up in making choices and decisions based on assumptions about what the person with dementia wants or needs. The creation of dependency by carers is a well known phenomenon where they take over all the lifestyle responsibilities for their relative with dementia. Although this can be an understandable response, the person with dementia experiences 'being done unto', and feels powerless and is often not listened to by carers.

Empowering the person with dementia is a complex process; it has implicit notions of power sharing and partnership, and tailoring supports to suit the preferences of the individual. It is a mistake to think that because a person with dementia may have lost their capacity to communicate adequately or has difficulties in coping with tasks of daily living that they are no longer social beings or have feelings.

An example of giving power over their daily circumstances back to the person with dementia is illustrated by Bob Davis in his book *My Journey into Alzheimer's Disease* (1989). He writes about how he felt things were becoming a problem to him when attempting to go to the toilet during the night. He would wake up feeling disoriented, anxious and fearful because he could not find the door out of the bedroom. One response to this problem could have been to provide a commode at the side of his bed. This would solve the immediate problem – the prevention of wet beds – and allowed him still to retain some control. However, such a response would do little for his self-esteem and ability to carry out a daily living task like everyone else. Given that control over one's life is part and parcel of feeling empowered, there perhaps is another solution which preserves dignity, and values the individual. The answer in Bob's situation was to form a path of rough textured carpet from his bedside to the bathroom. By standing on the rough carpet in his bare feet he received a tactile response which assisted his orientation. Bob was empowered. He retained control, decision making and, most important, his personal privacy and self-esteem by a fairly simple solution. More important, his limited retained abilities were used to work out an acceptable strategy rather than have his doctor focus on the deficits.

A major obstacle to the person with dementia retaining personal empowerment relates to their knowledge about what's happening to them. Often there is a conspiracy of silence about the fact that they have dementia, from workers and carers alike. They feel unable to talk about the illness for fear of causing upset and undue anxiety. So although the person with dementia, particularly in the early stages, may sense something is wrong no one explains things. One project leader of an extra care housing complex has a policy of discussing with the tenants that they have dementia. She explains to them on an individual basis what dementia is and why they are a tenant in the project. Responses may vary from the person who becomes upset and tearful, to the person who responds by saying 'There's nothing wrong with my memory' or 'I don't feel ill'. The importance of this approach is that it allows the care staff to begin at the point of the tenant's present understanding. The workers can then provide information, counselling and support so that the person regains a sense of being treated and valued as a unique individual. Empowerment for the person with dementia may not always have tangible outcomes other than the person feeling better in themselves or through a validation approach coming to terms with some past life crisis.

In striving to assist the person with dementia lead as normal a life as possible, consideration has to be given to the retained abilities and skills they have. Rather than focus on the deficits that the person might demonstrate, help the individual with dementia focus on what they still can do for themselves, and bring in supports appropriate to their level of functioning. Undoubtedly this is a balancing act for social workers! Empowerment is significantly different in that it begins by adopting a position whereby the problem definition is in terms of the user's understanding.

EMPOWERING CARERS

A carer who attended the training course related an incident when he contacted a social worker to arrange for his mother to be admitted for an overnight stay to a local residential home. The worker visited when the carer was not at home, questioned the mother, made an assessment, contacted the doctor and arranged for the carer's mother to be admitted to the assessment ward of the local hospital for two weeks' respite. Whilst this might have seemed an appropriate response to the worker the carer experienced a loss of power and control over his situation. This led to mistrust, confrontation and a feeling of guilt on the part of the carer. This carer may not have known what empowerment actually meant for him, but did know that in his situation he did not feel in control, neither were his wishes or ability to cope considered. Just think: if you are a customer of a large department store, and intend to buy something, what rights and service would you expect that would empower you? Take a few minutes to think about this before you read on.

I certainly would want a choice of merchandise, quality goods which were value for money. But I also would want the staff to be knowledgable about any enquiries I might have, to give me information, and to deal with me fairly in an individual manner. I most definitely would not want to be pressured and should be allowed to change my mind without fear of repercussion. Contained in all my wants and expectations is the notion that I am retaining control over my situation, so that I might express my individuality in the manner I choose.

If you took time to consider seriously that shopping scenario, what you will have realised is that our empowerment is dependent on the shop assistant's values, beliefs and attitudes and how he or she interprets the store policy for giving customer satisfaction, which might be seen as their philosophy of care. The maxim 'the customer is always right!' is, perhaps, a burden that shop assistants could do without. However, our expectations and attitude towards the shop assistant as a customer do not occur in a vacuum but maybe a result of previous experience in that particular shop, or based on what we have heard about the shop from others. This illustration can be used to emphasise some crucial factors concerning empowerment.

Having choices depends on recognising that other options exist (the selection of merchandise). But choosing a product will be dependent on what we think our need is and if there is more than one suitable product. We may therefore need to consider the pros and cons of a particular article and may also need to have someone help us decide. However, if we are spending our money then our wishes, and what we ultimately want will remain firmly in our control. The experience of many carers is that caring for their relative with dementia often means that things are out with their control.

As dementia affects the coping skills of their relative, this can result in them having to withdraw from normal daily activities. Their daily routine has to revolve around the caring tasks for their relative. Not only do carers talk about feeling a sense of isolation they also relate the pressures and stresses of coping with the effects of dementia on the relative, particularly if the individual ceases to be able to have sensible conversation. Mr B cared for his 78-year-old wife and said that all the communication that occurred between them was her repeating everything he said. He experienced a sense of frustration, particularly as she also confused night and day and wanted to be awake during the night. He felt a sense of guilt that he could not do more, yet did not know who to go to for help. Significantly, he wanted help, but not charity, wanted respite but on his terms, and wanted support that his wife would accept. It was for such reasons that a training course was set up for carers with the intention of providing support to them in their caring task.

What follows is a description of work undertaken in October 1991 with carers of people with dementia and representatives of health, social work and voluntary agencies. These people came together for two days and shared training sessions which had been set up with the explicit purpose of empowering carers. The work was subsequently researched two months later to identify whether there had been any significant impact on the carers coping. As will be shown there were clear outcomes, in that carers felt empowered.

TRAINING PROJECT

The rationale for the project centred around four themes:

1. That the work would enable a greater understanding between health and social work staff and carers.

2. That it would lead to a shared understanding which would lead to a more responsive service.

3. That it would provide education and knowledge about dementia and information about resources.

4. That it might help identify how services could be developed in line with community care legislation (Adams, Chapman, Farnase 1992).

Consequently, these statements became translated into the following aims:

1. To provide information and knowledge for professionals and carers about dementia so that they might be enabled to give effective stress-free support to people with dementia.

2. To raise awareness of professionals of the ways in which they might support carers of people with dementia.

3. To facilitate a locally based inter-disciplinary approach to the needs of carers of people with dementia.

4. To evaluate the effectiveness of the approach in terms of training experience and impact on service delivery.

Inviting the carers

Contact was made by personal invitation to those carers already known to the health and social work departments. Some carers were visited and invited after having explained to them the purpose of the training. Thirty-five carers were sent invitations, but only thirteen attended the sessions. A special lunchtime presentation was organised for all local professionals to attend and it was asked that a representative number opt to attend. Ten workers attended.

The training

The format for the training sessions was based on a knowledge of matters for which carers continually requested help. A two day programme was then devised which gave information about dementia, allowed time for carers and professionals to work together to share concerns and perceptions, identified local resources, explained care in the community legislation, and offered practical advice to carers about managing problem behaviour, continence management and welfare rights.

The trainers who carried out this project adopted a participative approach, allowing as much time as possible for discussion and dialogue around the topic areas. The intention was not to enter into a problem solving exercise, but rather to acknowledge and hear the concerns of carers and attempt to tailor the sessions accordingly. By virtue of professional staff also experiencing the same training sessions it was hoped that a spin off would be a greater understanding of the carers' situations whilst demystifying for carers the sometimes unclear roles of professionals.

One particular session highlighted the difference between the concerns of carers and the professionals' perceptions of carers' problems. The session involved all professionals discussing what they considered to be priority needs of the carers. At the same time the carers were discussing what were their main needs. Each group was provided with paper to list the needs in order of priority arising from their discussions. It was not surprising to learn that both carers and the professionals had similar lists of needs, but there was a variance in order of importance. Carers regarded practical help and advice about issues such as continence management and benefits as a high priority. Professionals perceived carers as requiring a charter of rights and, in their list of priorities, practical issues were rated as of a lower importance. This only indicates that if professionals are serious about empowering people then they cannot make assumptions based on their experience but require to talk and listen to carers.

The requirement that social service departments and health authorities enter into a consultation process with users has, I suspect and know from experience, little to do with empowerment. There is often little notion of power sharing but rather the expectation that the consultation will confirm already existing departmental plans. The baseline remains if professionals control budgets and access to resources then they will be reluctant to see that eroded in any way, despite what the legislation may state. The other problem is that users might request services which providers have ranked as being of a lower priority. The training again served to show this, particularly when discussing the very practical provision of incontinence pads. The adviser leading the session admitted that their stack of pads were not as good as the ones provided by hospitals, as these were more expensive. Although more effective for the person with dementia the community care budgets could not stretch to the hospital type, so the carers had to cope with second best.

Evaluation

An evaluation was carried out at the end of each two day session and an immediate reaction from all those involved was that the experience had been extremely useful. Professional workers talked about gaining insights into the needs of carers. Carers talked about, for the first time, being given clear information about dementia. Carers also began to understand and recognise the different roles that the various professionals undertook. The practical advice sessions were regarded as being particularly helpful.

Two months later

A researcher was employed to interview all the participants of the training and the outcomes were recorded by means of a questionnaire. Given that the intention had been to empower the carers, had this occurred?

Outcomes

The outcomes for carers highlighted the following:

1. The content of the training reflected what carers wanted to know.

2. The participative approach allowed carers to share experiences with professionals and allowed for an element of problem solving.

3. The confidence and self-esteem of the carers had been enhanced by being given special support via training.

4. Important practical advice was given which provided the carers with ideas about what resources and help was available.

5. Carers felt important because someone cared enough to provide a training experience.

6. The training provided an exchange of views and opinions in a relatively safe environment.

As a special project this approach of using training sessions as means of providing carer support for those involved achieved its original intentions. 'Carers felt more in control of their situation because of having gained new knowledge' (Adams, Chapman and Farnase 1992).

The outcomes for professionals were as follows:

1. All were enthusiastic about the shared training approach, as they had learned more of the role of the carer.

2. Initial perceptions of carers' needs altered as a result of workers gaining new insights into the stresses and burdens associated with caring.

3. The training course had met workers expectations and indications from some workers was that the course had been of direct benefit in helping them plan a quality service.

4. Most professionals felt that the course had not raised any service expectations which could not be met in practice.

5. All professionals felt that they were more aware of carers' requirements and need for support, based on a greater range of alternative options being on offer.

SUMMARISING THE ISSUES

Empowering users is not an easy task. To enable people to master their own environment and achieve what they want for themselves involves workers in reframing their ideas about the essence of the social work task. To create an empowering relationship involves recognising the unique life experience of individuals, and valuing the contribution they can make to resolving a particular need. The idea of power sharing and partnership has implications for workers about how they intervene in situations, particularly when making an assessment of need for the person with dementia. This means being prepared to spend time, however little, communicating so as to allow them to understand what's happening and to express some opinion. It also means listening to the significant others in the situation who may not always be relatives. Such information from the network of supporters undoubtedly often provides valuable help. What others may see as appropriate may bear little relation to what the person with dementia understands their problem to be, and therefore a solution which satisfies their wishes.

If the person with dementia is to continue living in their own home, and is to have individual self determination, then the worker has to allow a degree of risk taking and adopt an enabling approach. This involves a degree of power sharing and partnership with the user; not taking over but utilising the retained abilities that the person with dementia has. So the worker might begin to act as a catalyst for individuals to achieve actions for themselves. The situation in reality could, perhaps, be better but as in the example of Bob Davies it seems important to consider strategies that maintain individuality and sense of control. This may be helping them work out solutions to particular difficulties as in the example of Bob Davis or enabling a choice to be presented so that a decision can be reached.

The example of the training for carers also brings some important points to our attention. The training was intended to be non-patronising in nature and create a sense of each carer having their experience valued. This was achieved by avoiding lecture-type presentations, using an informal room layout and encouraging discussion. However, the message is just as valid for community based workers.

Another important factor in the training was that of not providing simple answers to complex problems and of recognising the many stresses involved in caring for someone with dementia. As has been mentioned in the chapter on groupwork, carers have an unremitting burden and their ability to cope is often dependent on the support available to them. Consequently, for the worker this requires a more creative approach to how and what resources are to be used. The carer requiring a break from the burden of caring may only want three or four hours a week, and not the two week block once every six months. Social workers have to engage in negotiation and partnership with both the carer and a manager of a care unit so that the carer feels and experiences being allowed to manage their situation. Empowerment begins with recognising the potential that people as individuals have to cope with situations, and allowing self determination.

As a professional worker what approach will you adopt with the next person with dementia and their carer? Will you adopt an enabling and power sharing relationship or will you take control and so foster dependency? Empowering the individual with dementia and/or carers inherently requires the worker to be aware of their differing needs and his or her personal value system.

REFERENCES

Adams, E., Chapman, A. and Farnase, R. (1992) *Carers and Professionals Together*. Stirling: Dementia Services Development Centre.

Clough, R. (1990) *Practice, Politics, and Power in Social Service Departments*. Aldershot: Avebury Gower Publishing.

Davis, B. (1989) *My Journey into Alzheimer's Disease*. Illinois: Tyndale House Publications.

Keiffer, C. (1984) Citizen Empowerment, A Developmental Perspective. *Prevention in Human Services* 3–201–226.

NHS and Community Care Act (1990) London: HMSO

Perlman, H.H. (1957) *Social Casework: A Problem-Solving Process*. Cambridge: Cambridge University Press.

Rowley, D. and Taylor, L. (1992) *Planning and Managing Community Care*. University of Dundee.

Simmons, C. and Parsons, R. (1983) Empowerment for Role Alternatives in Adolescence. *Adolescence* 18 (69) 193–200.

Tossell, D. and Webb, R. (1986) *Inside the Caring Services*. London: Edward Arnold.

Turner, J.B. (1977) *Encyclopedia of Social Work*. Washington: National Association of Social Workers.

Wolfensberger, W. (1972) *The Principle of Normalisation in Human services*. Toronto: National institute of mental retardation.

POINTS FOR DISCUSSION

1. What do you personally understand by the concept 'empowerment?' What might empowerment mean for a client in the early stages of dementia?

2. What difficulties have you experienced, or can you envisage, in empowering clients generally in social work practice? What methods are appropriate to tackling such difficulties?

3. Discuss the relationship between empowerment and offering choices to people with dementia and to their carers.

4. Does the Care in the Community legislation legitimate and/or inhibit, choice and empowerment to clients with dementia?

5. Discuss the value of the example of a training course for carers as a means to promote empowerment.

6. Do you agree that the choice for you as a social worker is between power-sharing or fostering dependency?

CHAPTER EIGHT

Assessment and Care Management of People with Dementia and their Carers

Katrina Myers and J. Crawford

In this chapter we will consider the process of assessment and care management and the experience of how this worked in one particular project, the Elderly People in the Community (EPIC) Project. We will illustrate this with a case study of a client who was involved in the Project.

THE TRADITIONAL VIEW OF ASSESSMENT

Assessment has, for many years, been the method used by professionals to determine whether people meet the criteria for a particular service. Different assessment formats exist, but essentially they all act as a 'sifting' process, by identifying those most vulnerable. The focus, therefore, was to use assessment as a gatekeeper to the resources, be it home help, meals on wheels and residential accommodation.

The emphasis of the National Health Services and Community Care Act is on moving away from this service-led assessment, where the assessor begins with a set of criteria for services and decides how the person fits in. This approach to assessment begins by taking a look at the needs of the individual. The assessment ensures that the individual client is placed at the centre of the process in order for their needs to be met. When dealing with someone with dementia, who may be disorientated of time and place, it is essential that they and their carers are placed at the centre of any assessment or care plan and that their wishes are taken into account at each decision being made. In this way, assessment and care management could help to improve the way we work with people with dementia and their carers.

THE COMPONENTS OF CARE MANAGEMENT

The idea of care management emerged in North America during the early 1970s and 1980s and in the UK as pilot projects in the late 1970s and 1980s. The components of care management, which is regarded as the core of good social work practice, include some of the following:

1. Assessment of need.

2. Delivery of care packages.

3. Review of the quality of care provided.

4. Reassessment of client needs.

The model used by any particular project or authority will be influenced by the kind of organisation, the particular needs of the client group and decisions about how the care manager relates to other professionals. There is no clear model which works particularly well with people with dementia and their carers. It can, however, be argued that any method of working which pays attention to individual needs in a complicated care situation will be experienced as a positive and helpful method so far as the client and the carer are concerned.

MODELS OF CARE MANAGEMENT

In an analysis of five UK case management projects, Beardshaw and Towell (1990) show us the variety of elements which are around for care management.[*] There can be very diverse factors such as numbers in case loads varying, the different background of care managers, the access to resources and the access to budgets.

Beardshaw and Towell discuss two broad models of care management: social entrepreneurship and service brokerage. Social entrepreneurship is close to the model used in EPIC, where the care manager had a notional budget set at two thirds of the cost of residential care. The role of the care manager was to bring together a network of help, formal and informal, to maintain the individual in the community. Existing services such as domiciliary home carers could be used or, alternatively, individual forms of support for a particular client could be developed.

---

[*] It should be noted that the term care management is now used in preference to 'case management' which was used in earlier projects.

Such an approach involves the care manager in adopting a coordinating and enabling role, with close links being formed with other professionals.

The service brokerage model places an emphasis on contracts between the client and the care manager with the care manager acting as an advocate for the client. Supports are organised in response to the individual needs.

There will be debates about who holds the budget, whether care management is a 'role' for the social worker or a 'task' within an existing role. The care management team may require to be comprised of joint social work and health personnel. This is particularly true with dementia where it is essential for health and social care to work in tandem.

EPIC PROJECT

The EPIC Project was set up in 1990 by Forth Valley Health Board and Central Regional Council Social Work Department. It ran for two years and was evaluated by the University of Stirling whose report is available for further study.

The project was based in Stirling Royal Infirmary and served the Stirling area. Its aim was to maintain vulnerable elderly people at home by developing the provision of effective domiciliary care and support for the client, in particular people with dementia and their carers. This was achieved through the introduction of a care management approach and the establishment of a multidisciplinary team of health and social work staff. It attempted to make the best of existing services by ensuring effective coordination and to promote the development of innovative forms of assistance. This process was based on a comprehensive needs assessment and the provision of individual care packages.

Care management in this project had four main aims:

1. To bring health and social care systems closer together in the care management team.

2. To devise common criteria for comprehensive multidisciplinary assessment.

3. To institute care planning on the basis of need and 'best provision' rather than for a pre-determined form of service.

4. To ensure coordination of services through a care manager.

Care managers completed a detailed assessment of day and night needs, devising individual care plans which were regularly monitored and reviewed. The care managers were able to control and deploy a devolved budget.

The team consisted of a project leader (social work background), a social worker, a community psychiatric nurse, an occupational therapist and a health visitor. Referrals were accepted from the local primary health care, social work teams and voluntary agencies. On occasion, referrals were accepted directly from the carer or the family. There were regular links with other identified social work and health personnel, including a geriatrician and psychogeriatrician. This group of professionals, known as the extended team, provided additional expertise upon which the care manager could draw.

An essential feature of the project was the recruitment and deployment of specially trained home carers, providing the kinds of personal care which might be given by a close relative, including dressing, washing, putting to bed, as well as some domestic tasks. This small group proved to be an essential factor in allowing a high degree of flexibility in the care provided. They were available at times which suited the situation, and could engage in a range of caring tasks.

Although the care management team was specialist, it worked closely and integrated its activities with the referring practitioners, sharing skills and resources and working across health/social work organisational boundaries.

For the purpose of the EPIC Project the care managers operated with a notional budget, which was set at two thirds of the cost of residential or hospital care. So, although the budget was not calculated on an individual client basis, it did reflect whether the client would have used hospital or residential care. At the time of referral to EPIC this budget figure was used to determine whether the cost of a proposed package of care would exceed the stipulated figure. If so, the client was not accepted onto the project and was referred to hospital or residential care.

Once a client was accepted by the project this cost was not a factor, although by use of a computer system which had details of costs for every unit of care, individual care plans were costed out on a weekly basis. So, if a client needed five days daycare, for example, this could be calculated and recorded on the care plan. The research will tell us how useful this exercise of the notional budget has been.

The project did have a devolved budget which was operated by the Project leader. The 'real' money enabled the project to employ and train their home carers, to buy time from Crossroads on a contractual basis and to buy extra home help time when this was necessary. The budget gave the project a real degree of flexibility in the development of care plans.

According to the Social Services Inspectorate and Social Work Services Group (1992) 'Care management is the process of tailoring services to individual needs. Assessment is an integral part of care management but it is only one of six core tasks that make up the whole process:

1. Publishing information.

2. Determining the level of assessment.

3. Assessing need.

4. Care planning.

5. Implementing the care plan.

6. Monitoring and review.'

We will use these six core tasks to structure the rest of the chapter and interweave the case study to illustrate the process.

PUBLISHING INFORMATION

It is thought that the information in this document should be comprehensive, assessable and accurate. Clients and carers will need different information at different times. For instance, in the early stages there will be a greater need for information about the disease, to forewarn the person and the carer of the future. At a later stage it might be more important for them to know about particular services or benefits available to them. It will be the responsibility of the care manager to be aware of all this information with which to enable the client to make informed choices about their care.

As dementia can leave families/carers feeling very isolated, it is helpful if ways can be found to make sure that all information is published in ways which are accessible. Often the strain of caring can hinder the individual from finding out what is available; the challenge will be in bringing the information to the carer and client. All information about services needs to be collated in a way which will make it available to the client, the carer and all professionals. The key person is often the GP, whose role can be essential in opening doors for the client. Any care manager will need to develop strong links with the health professions to ensure good collaboration. The doctor's surgery or the health clinic will be an excellent source of information for the client, a good point for disseminating information.

This will be a difficult task, requiring skills which do not traditionally relate to social work practice. In the past, social work organisations have tended not to advertise or disseminate information, perhaps from a fear of being inundated with demands for help! Other issues arise around the format of the information, the use of jargon and versions available in different languages to ensure access to a wide range of people.

One of the strong themes of care in the community is the empowerment of the client. The opportunity to make informed choice is one way of shifting power from the 'expert' to the 'client', thus, making real attempts to publicise information which will help people make decisions about what will improve their situation.

Putting power back into the hands of the carer is particularly essential in relation to those with dementia. Marshall (1990) poses the question 'Does "community care" for this group have any meaning?' and draws attention to their vulnerability and the threat to their rights as individuals: '... they may be considered to be unable to have a say in matters that affect their physical safety... anyone needing help cannot freely exercise choice unless they receive adequate support...' The care manager can provide the client with information which allows her to make a choice from a range of services available to meet her needs. The carer may be the main focus for communication between one person with dementia and the care manager. The word 'support' could include information and advice.

Local authorities and health boards are now bound by the National Health Service and Community Care Act to publish community care plans. They are expected to develop a system of consultation which enables everyone with any contact with their services to comment on and contribute to the formulation of the strategic plan. The care manager with his/her direct contact with the carer and client will be able to feed into this system.

DETERMINING THE LEVEL OF ASSESSMENT/TARGETING

In Kent (Challis and Davies 1986) and Gateshead (Challis *et al.* 1990) case finding was targeted at the group of elderly people at risk of being admitted to residential care. In EPIC a combination of the following criteria were used to determine who would be able to use this service:

- age 70+
- were physically very disabled
- had mild to moderate dementia
- were in receipt of or in need of multiple community services
- were in receipt of a high intensity single community service
- were being cared for by families under considerable stress or burden
- were at risk of needing longterm institutional care

These were people with complex needs, requiring more than a one-off assessment leading to an allocation of a resource. This would be a 'complex' case which demanded an approach which allowed for time to be spent in assessing the needs in the situation. Referrals were made to the project on a screening form, with ten questions (Appendix 8.1), which could be scored on a scale of one to ten, indicating the level of need (Lutz *et al.* 1989). The referral form was most useful when completed by someone who knew the client, thus providing sufficient information to determine the complexity of the situation and inform the decision about whether or not a care manager becomes involved.

Judy Renshaw (1988) summarises: 'The main aim of case management is to meet the needs of clients in the most suitable and individualised way, rather than to fit people into the standard services which happen to be available... Working from a central coordinating point increases the likelihood of equitable treatment, and good communications should improve access'. She further says:

> Achieving fair and equitable distribution of resources requires that similar cases should be treated in similar ways (and, of course, that different needs receive appropriately different service packages). This implies a thorough and competent assessment which is well-standardised, so that the same criteria are applied to all cases at different points in time and in different locations.

The Scottish Office Guidelines to Care Management (1992) suggest that social work authorities should exercise their lead responsibility in community care by negotiating a set of minimum requirements for referral information:

> The aim of the initial information gathering is to establish as quickly and as sensitively as possible the *urgency, level and complexity of needs* to inform the allocation decision. This will determine the speed and type of assessment response.

In our case study, which is typical of many in the community, Mrs X was referred by her GP. Aged seventy five, she is a widow on her own. The referral describes her as having poor mobility, forgetful and requiring more help to care for herself. At first glance it looks as if she has a number of services and is being well provided for. In fact, many of the services were inappropriate to her needs and had broken down. The list of services and supports included home help, Crossroads, health visitor, meals on wheels, social worker, GP, daycare, carer (niece), carer (brother) and Mobile Emergency Care Services (MECS).

None of the professionals involved had made a comprehensive assessment of her total needs. As a result, the complexity of her circumstances did not come to light until there was a crisis. This crisis developed when her brother, her main carer who lived two streets away, died and left her without someone in regular contact to care for her.

ASSESSING NEED

In considering the role of social work in the assessment process, it will be easy to assume that we know all about assessment. Social workers have been making assessments for many years, so what is new? We would like to suggest that we need to reconsider our approach to assessment.

> The need to move towards a more genuinely holistic model of assessment where client and carer wishes are central and which has as its goal the identification of a range of appropriate supports for clients, rather than standard service packages, is widely recognised. (Beardshaw and Towell 1990)

The challenge of social work in the new era of community care is to make 'needs led' assessments and move away from assessment for services. This is not easy as the pragmatic social worker is bound to look at any situation in relation to services which already exist. It needs a change of organisation, access to budget and some space in workload to enable the development of an approach which includes a range of flexible services. It is preferable to think about a 'needs led' approach which is informed by current services but which can be flexible enough to identify and assist in the development of new services. It is not practical to 'throw out' all existing services, but it is possible to drop some of the thinking which prevents an imaginative use of these resources.

In the EPIC Project a standardised form was developed (Lutz *et al.* 1989) to provide a multi-dimensional assessment of needs. We will refer to this in the next few pages.

Different issues related to the assessment of someone with dementia

It is impossible to think about assessment of someone with dementia without looking at the issue of diagnosis. Early diagnosis can be the starting point for the person with dementia, the carers and the family. It can be the point at which people begin to come to terms with the situation. There are mixed views about the impact of the diagnosis of dementia. In terms of provision of help, the diagnosis is the necessary key to open the door to sources of support and practical help. Without a diagnosis there will be an uphill struggle to gain access to benefits. The diagnosis can be a very difficult, painful process and it may be the first time that someone acknowledges that something is wrong. Regardless of the stage of dementia, the difficulties about diagnosis will exist.

In terms of skills, the care manager will need to develop very sensitive listening and communication skills at this stage. This will allow an atmosphere wherein the impact of the diagnosis can be handled and explored to enable the person and the carer to begin to accept the situation. If sensitivity is not present the person with dementia and the carer may feel abandoned and let down. The most important factor in assessment is knowledge of the illness, what it is, the progress of the disease, the effect on the individual and the impact on the family.

> The priority requirement for assessment staff will be an in depth understanding of the needs associated with particular user groups and a knowledge of the range of services and community resources available to meet those needs. (SSI and SWSG 1992)

In our case study there was a diagnosis, but this may not have been communicated to everyone involved with Mrs X; for example, The Mobile Emergency Care Service (MECS) is not usually available to a person with dementia as it requires an understanding of how the alarm system operates. We were unsure from the referral if Mrs X had in fact developed dementia since being connected up to this alarm call service.

Caring for someone with dementia can result in many needs for the carer and for the person. Any assessment of need may be limited by the client's inability to participate in the assessment process. The challenge lies in finding a way to communicate with the carer and the person to try to discern their views on needs. When the person is no longer able to communicate, we must be very clear about the underlying philosophy of working with people with dementia. This is underpinned by an attempt to improve or at least maintain a good quality of life for the client and the carer.

The concepts of dignity, rights and choice, where possible, must inform social work practice with this client group. An attempt to understand the person's lifestyle, and their likes and dislikes, and their past activities, will help the care manger translate these concepts into practice. The form used in the EPIC Project encourages the care manager to discuss things directly with the client. It is essential to always attempt this, thus avoiding the temptation to ignore the client who has difficulty in communicating.

How is the actual process of assessment different? In the first stage, in response to the referral, access may be difficult. The care manager may choose to invite the referrer to go with them or to be in the house when they call. This acknowledges the potential for anxiety in the person with dementia if they do not know the care manager. To be introduced by a known person can make a big difference. Access can be more difficult if there is no carer; the assessor must be imaginative in how they gain access to the person. Remember that the person with dementia, living on their own, may live in a state of anxiety with an impaired ability to relate to new people.

Time may also be a factor which is different. As the person with dementia may be difficult to communicate with, time and patience may be needed to build up a full picture of the situation. In the EPIC Project the care management role was the main role for all the project staff. This allowed them time to concentrate on the assessment task and allow the time needed for communication. It might be essential to have someone present who knows the person, to assist the care manager with the assessment. If there is no carer, no obvious family or friendly supporter, the assessor will have to spend time with the person, gaining their trust. At this stage the assessor will be looking for the pieces of the jigsaw. It might help to involve anyone who has contact: carer, friend, family, neighbours. Any other professionals' knowledge and viewpoint will be useful in the assessment process. It is usually a good idea to seek the person's permission before contacting other people, the question will arise as to how informed this permission will be. On balance it will be helpful to make a real attempt to gain permission to make yourself understandable to the person with dementia.

N.B. *If there is a main carer, it may be possible to use this relationship to enable a full picture to be put together.* The quality of the relationship will be the deciding factor in how useful this contact is. If the relationship is poor, this may well be a source of difficulty and the care plan may include some work on this relationship. If the relationship is a positive one, the carer may act as a channel of communication for the person with dementia. When we look at the analysis of the diaries using network analysis, it is apparent that Mrs Smith is totally dependent on her daughter for maintaining any communication with the outside world. This shows up the potential for non-communication for the person with dementia who lives on her own. In our case study, Mrs X is an example where the care manager develops the role as the person who acts as a channel between her and the outside world.

It will be of considerable importance to be mindful of the person's life history as this could inform the assessor about previous personality and experiences. Often knowledge of the person's past can lead to a greater understanding of how they are in the present. Part of the care plan may include the development of a life story book in which information about the person's past will be important for use in the future (Myers 1991). The more detailed a knowledge and understanding of the person's past, the more flexible current carers can be in how they work with the individual. This is considerably different from working with clients who do not have dementia; the nature of the detail of past history will be different. It might help, for instance, to know details of each house lived in, each job worked in and the 'normal' routines of the person's life.

Perhaps more so than with other client groups, involvement of the carer must be a part of the formal process. In the EPIC Project, there is a separate section of the assessment document seeking information about the carer's own situation. This can give some indication of the stress involved in the particular situation which might be an important factor in the process. In this part of the assessment form, the subjects covered include living arrangements, financial costs, the effect of caring on privacy, any tensions caused by caring, the carer's self-reported health, attitude to caring and help. This puts the carer at the centre, along with the person with dementia, fully acknowledging their importance in the whole situation.

In working with this client group it is advisable to concentrate on what the person can do; on retained skills rather than on deficits. Taking a more positive approach may help the carer retain some interest and commitment. If a more positive approach is taken, the person with dementia is more likely to respond and work with you to retain skills. Depending on the effect of the 'caring task' on the carer, work may need to be done directly with them in helping them develop coping strategies.

The assessment format

The question of assessment forms is always a difficult one to answer. There are arguments for and against the use of a set format or questionnaire. At this time, there is not a comprehensive, all-purpose form which the Dementia Services Development Centre can recommend. Most authorities develop their own, to suit their particular need. Our only plea is that assessors use them only as an aid to, or as part of the assessment process. In this we acknowledge that many forms can be used to great effect, but these must complement the assessor's skills and knowledge of the assessment process. In the process of concentrating on the assessment form, the assessor who is under pressure may forget to act as a human being and respond to the immediate needs of the person to be listened to and included in the process.

The EPIC Project developed a comprehensive assessment form which is too large to quote in full, but the following is a list of headings used: 'Housing, financial needs, accidents and emergencies, physical health, mental health, help and support received, managing daily living – seven days in the week and carer assessment form'. There is no specific section to assess how the person is affected by dementia but questions are used throughout to ascertain its effect on specific difficulties; for instance, under financial needs the question included is 'Does the applicant have difficulty in handling money and understanding his/her financial affairs?' In the section on Mental Health there are questions about disorientation, memory, behaviour and mood. All of these could indicate dementia and how it affects the person's daily living. This format helps to organise the information required and includes the client's opinion wherever possible, including the question 'What can be done to alleviate the problem?'.

In using this form, a number of skills will come in to play. The assessor will find ways of compensating for the person's particular disability. This will not be easy, as progress might be slow. Counselling skills will enable the assessor to listen to those involved, to encourage any communication, regardless of their limitations. The challenge is not to try to solve problems at the beginning, but to use our counselling skills to understand the situation from the client and carer's point of view. By placing the person with dementia at the centre, alongside the carer, it will be more likely that the assessment will highlight real needs.

One very challenging aspect of working with people with dementia is our need to develop very sensitive enabling communication skills. An ability to explain the process to the client and the carer, verbally and in writing will be of great benefit in this process. As the person with dementia may not be easily understandable, the care manager's needs for empathy, patience and awareness of emotional responses will be apparent. The switch, subtle but difficult, will be in the responsibility for the communication, so that it is less of an even, two-way process and there is more responsibility on the care manager to develop the communication. Through competent communication skills, the assessor's skills will be needed to enable the person with dementia to communicate to the best of their ability. By actively listening and engaging with the carer, the worker will discover what can be done to enable the carer to carry on. It is right to remember that as the person with dementia becomes less able to communicate with us, we have to become more skilled at communicating with them.

Skills involved in liaison and joint working will be very useful. This begins with working with the client and carer, as partners, and then includes working with other colleagues in the social work department and in the health professions. In the field of dementia the edges between social care and health care become blurred and it will be invariably be helpful to include other professionals' knowledge and opinions in the assessment. As assessment merges into care planning, advocacy and negotiation skills will become more relevant.

In conclusion, therefore, the essentials for a full needs-led assessment can be summed up by stating that the assessor must have an up-to-date knowledge of dementia, must be prepared to work along with the client, the carer, and any other relevant persons and must allow enough time to build up a full picture of the whole situation. The care manager will need to look out for the 'ripple in the pool' effect of dementia. The person with dementia is sometimes the stone which starts the ripple, but the effects reach out in wider and wider circles, affecting many people in different ways. Part of the assessment will include the effect of the ripple on the wider circle of family and friends.

The emergency situation often prevents careful, full assessment being made. However, with the use of these skills outlined and a sound underlying philosophy this need not be lost. The monitoring and reviewing stages of care planning will compensate for any gaps in the assessment stage.

Before moving on to the next stage it might be useful to look at Mrs X by the end of the assessment, but before the care plan is put together (see diagram in Appendix 8.2). It became apparent that Mrs X was more dependent on her brother than anyone had known. This is often the case, where the carer gradually increases their attention and support to compensate for the deterioration in the person with dementia. The carer can thus mask the gradual onset of the illness and the extent of the care required.

The distant carer, Mrs X's niece, found herself in the role of the main carer. Quite overwhelmed by the situation, she was unable to contribute much direct care because of her own family and work commitments and she lived some distance away. She was anxious to respect her aunt's wish to remain in her own home. A number of the services were found to be unsuitable. Mrs X could no longer use MECS, the alarm system. Day care had stopped; no one really knew why. The social worker had left the department and had not been replaced. Meals on wheels were still delivered but were not being eaten. A psychogeriatric assessment had been made a year before, with no follow up. It was clear that a re-assessment was necessary.

CARE PLANNING

Central to the purpose of care management is that it allows vulnerable people who would otherwise have little control over their circumstances to maximise their independence and gain control over their care.

Mrs X had been very clear that she wanted to remain in her own home. The EPIC Project aimed to maintain vulnerable elderly people at home. These two aims could be achieved through the implementation of a care plan. Where there are several services and workers involved, the person with dementia and their carer must know the name of the person in the coordinating role, so that they know exactly to whom to turn if there is any change in the situation. The care manager has to be seen as the route into a network of services, not another service with which the carer or the client has to do battle. This relationship begins at the time of assessment and develops throughout the care management process. The role of the care manager is clearly that of coordinator and communicator to all those involved.

Bland *et al.* (1992) point out that, generally, elderly people have low expectations for themselves and tend not to mention difficulties; they frequently define problems in terms of their often very partial knowledge of what services are available and define needs according to a very restricted definition of services. The role of the care manger includes looking beyond these low expectations, and encouraging the person to state their needs. The care manager provides the client and carer with consumer choice.

> The more comprehensive the practitioner's knowledge at this stage, the more imaginative they can be in making relevant and cost-effective use of available resources. (Scottish Office 1992)

As we have already stated, access to a budget is an important factor in care planning. This is not to say that these care managers have unlimited scope (they must at all times be aware of the limits within which their agency can work) but it does allow for imaginative care planning. In Mrs X's case, for example, the care manager was able to set up a care plan which introduced a home carer and also a contract with Crossroads, both of which were paid for out of the devolved budget to provide a service which was otherwise unobtainable.

Initially a care plan was drawn up to cover mornings (dressing and breakfast), lunch times and evenings, seven days a week, using the home help, Crossroads care attendant and a home carer (care being taken to use people already known to Mrs X and to introduce new workers gradually). The care manager negotiated the continuing involvement of the community nurse.

Mrs X's niece was relieved of the worry of the daily difficulties presented by her aunt and, in consultation with the care manager, she took responsibility for the management of her aunt's finances.

Designing the care plan was taken at Mrs X's own pace and the care manager was able to work with her, accepting her strong wish to stay at home and find ways to meet her needs in a way which was acceptable to her. Great care was taken to build on Mrs X's relationships with people, to minimise disruption. Any change was seen as a potential source of anxiety to her so caution was to be taken with this.

IMPLEMENTING THE CARE PLAN

Frequently, care managers will interweave the formal and informal inputs into the care plan, often reordering existing arrangements into a more effective package. This sometimes involves long and hard negotiations with all parties concerned, in order that it is clearly agreed who does what.

Services may have to be provided in a more flexible way that is more appropriate to the individual needs of the person with dementia and their carer, and the care manager has to introduce changes sensitively. In our case study, the rapidly progressing dementia of Mrs X made it necessary to design a complex care package, but at the same time keep unfamiliar faces to a minimum. The home help was, therefore, paid as a home carer out of hours (out of the Project's devolved budget) for some of the evenings, and the Crossroads care attendant was contracted to cover lunchtimes and weekends. Despite a big increase in input, only one new worker was introduced initially: the EPIC home carer.

In working with the person with dementia, we have to remember the potential for change. In this case there was deterioration due to dementia and over the period of time a number of changes were made to the care plan. Eventually a re-assessment was made by the psychogeriatrician which resulted in Mrs X's attendance at the psychiatric day hospital five days a week. Some other changes included:

- bringing in the physiotherapist to show the home carers how to assist Mrs X with dressing and using her zimmer
- laundry service for bedding and clothes
- contact with health visitor re medication
- rearrangement of plans when, for instance, Mrs X had an appointment at the Eye Clinic or when the doctor visited re Attendance Allowance Assessment to ensure that she was available and someone was with her
- negotiating with day hospital staff about the management of Mrs X's poor hygiene

The care manager retained the role of communicating with home care organiser, GP, day hospital, community nursing team, the carer and anyone else with any interest in Mrs X.

The assessment and care plan placed Mrs X and her carer firmly at the centre, supported by the care manager. The care manager was able to share the responsibility with the main carer, taking away the day-to-day responsibility for Mrs X's care and safety. At the same time the carer maintained an important role in her aunt's care.

This work took place over a lengthy period and as Mrs X's dementia progressed it became apparent that she would not always be maintained at home. Eventually she accepted respite care in the local psychiatric hospital and thereafter agreed to be admitted on a permanent basis. This could only have been achieved through the work of the care manager who provided her with a safe environment which preserved a quality of life for her within her home until her needs for longterm care necessitated her admission. Although hard to prove, it seems that the relationship and trust built up with the care manager enabled Mrs X to accept a move which, 15 months before, would have been impossible for her.

In Mrs X's case the care plan was implemented as timeously as possible, and care was taken to fit in with the person's pace and lifestyle. The dignity of the person with dementia and his/her carer should be preserved in the way that assistance is given. Their wishes should always be central to the plan and they should be consulted in any changes or adjustments which are made; they must feel in control of the situation. Very often when the care manager is seen by the carer to take responsibility for the care plan, the carer may come back into a situation with more energy and commitment than before.

On the other hand, effective and sensitive work with carers is complicated by the fact that the interests of the carers and their needs are sometimes at odds with the interests and needs of the elderly person for whom they care. It may even be necessary to introduce another person to act for either party in any dispute or clash of interest. The development of advocacy as a way of working with people with dementia and their carers will be needed as care in the community maintains people at home for longer periods and the potential for clashes of interest increase. There may be a role for another colleague from the health services or a voluntary organisation to work with one of the parties.

MONITORING AND REVIEW

In some ways the care plan can never be set in stone as the situation will change, as shown in our case study. Beardshaw and Towell (1990) have pointed out that, where there are several services provided to an elderly person, monitoring and review arrangements often fail to be clarified. Before the development of a care plan, in our case study, meals on wheels and the MECS alarm were no longer appropriate, day care had broken down, the social worker had left, and the main carer died suddenly; exacerbating an already fraught situation. If a care manager had been involved from the outset on a continuing basis, the services would have been relevant, and the carer's death less traumatic in terms of the old lady's safety and well-being. Look at Appendix 8.3 to see a diagram of the changed situation when the Care Package is implemented.

Monitoring may be carried out in a number of ways, depending on the complexity of the situation; home visits, telephone calls, letters, inter-agency consultations, observations, and so forth. It is naturally important that the daily pattern of living of the person with dementia should be disrupted as little as possible.

> Whereas each contributor has a responsibility for the quality of their own input, the monitoring practitioner is accountable for the total quality of care as it is experienced by the user. (Scottish Office 1992)

This seems straightforward, but in practice the care manager may have to negotiate and press for all the contributors to maintain their input and commitment to the plan. This assumes a measure of experience, confidence and maturity in the care manager, whatever the model of care management employed.

A review should be held at intervals agreed by all parties concerned, and need not necessitate meetings of *all* involved, which are difficult to arrange and expensive of practitioner's time. The care manager usually, of course, consults with the other workers, carers and the user, to get an up-to-date picture of their opinions. Experience on the EPIC Project has shown that it is often helpful and appropriate to hold a review in the user's home, when they can participate. The care manager will always need to use his/her own judgement as to whether this is acceptable or would perhaps be too overwhelming.

In the case of dementia, where the disease progresses and there is sometimes an increase in the element of risk in maintaining the person at home, there is a great need for the monitoring and reviewing process to happen at regular intervals. Where risk is involved, monitoring alerts the care manager to any changes and the review is a mechanism for sharing the anxieties and keeping everyone to a consistent, shared strategy of care.

The carer and the person with dementia should have the confidence that the care manager will respond to any situation; this is basic to good care management practice. This is not to say that the care manager can necessarily provide a solution.

CONCLUSION

It is clear to the authors of this chapter that a system of assessment and care management can lead to an improved quality of life for the person with dementia and their carers. By taking an example of a project whose aim was to maintain vulnerable elderly people at home, at least 50 per cent of whom were people with dementia, it is clear that care management as a method of working is one to be encouraged. In our case study we saw how a number of services were provided for a client, who previously had had no full assessment of need, no coordination of services and no means to monitor and review. The result was a waste of resources, potentially a lack of support for the main carer and a crisis when the carer died unexpectedly. Without the EPIC Project with its assessment and care management service, Mrs X may well have had to leave home at crisis point. As a result of an appropriate coordinated package of care which suited her needs and allowed her to stay at home, Mrs X's quality of life was initially improved and then maintained for some time.

This was a very complex case which demanded a flexible response.

The care manager was able to coordinate this response. Students might like to ask themselves the question: What quality of life would Mrs X have achieved without this intervention?

REFERENCES

Beardshaw, V. and Towell, D. (1990) *Assessment and Case Management: Implications for the Implementation of Caring for People*. London: Kings Fund Institute.

Bland, R. and Bland, R. (1990) *Working Paper: Measuring Quality of Care in Old People's Homes*. Stirling: University of Stirling.

Bland, R.G., Hudson, H.M. and Dobson, B.M. (1992) *The EPIC Evaluation: Interim Report*. Stirling: University of Stirling.

Challis, D. and Davies, B. (1986) *Case Management in Community Care*. Southampton: Gower.

Challis *et al.* (1990) *Case Management in Social and Health Care: The Gateshead Community Care Scheme*. Personal Social Services Research Unit, Kent. Canterbury: University of Kent.

Lutz, B. in association with Bland, R., Cheetham, J. and Yelloly, M. (1989) *The Report of the Development and Testing of Screening and Assessment Instruments*. Stirling: Social Work Research Centre.

Marshall, M. (1990) (ed) *Working with Dementia: Guidelines for Professionals*. Birmingham: Venture Press.

Myers, K. (1991) *Life Story Books*. Stirling: Dementia Services Development Centre.

Renshaw, J. (1988) Care in the community: individual care planning and care management. *British Journal of Social Work* Vol 18. Oxford: University Press.

SSI and SWSG (1992) *Care Management and Assessment: Practitioners Guide*. London: HMSO.

Scottish Office (1992) *Guidelines to Care Management*. Edinburgh: HMSO.

Appendix 8.1: EPIC Project – Referral Form

Person completingName of person referring Form (tick one)

- [ ] GP
- [ ] Social worker
- [ ] Occupational therapist
- [ ] Home help organiser
- [ ] Community nurse/ health visitor
- [ ] Other

Address

Date of referral _____   Tel no _____

Name of client _____

Social work (CIS) number _____   Sex [ ]

Date of birth _____

Address _____   Tel no _____

Instructions for Completing the Form

You will notice that the initial question (see inside) asks if the older person lives alone or with other/s.

Alone – If 'alone' then put a tick in the box and tick marital status.

'Alone' in this instance means living permanently alone; if, at the time you are filling out the form, a person who usually lives with an other/s is temporarily alone (the spouse/ partner/relative/friend etc with whom s/he lives is, for example, in hospital and expected to return home) still regard this person as 'living with other/s'.

With Other/s – If the older person lives 'with other/s' enter a tick in the box, tick with whom the older person lives.

To Answer Question – Simply circle the correct response 'Yes', 'No', or 'DK' (don't know).

Comments and Suggestions – Please do add any essential information in the spaces provided that you think should be known about the older person which the questions do not cover and which would be essential in evaluating the 'at risk' status.

Please add any additional information here about the older person which you feel is essential for evaluating 'at risk' status. For example, blindness, loss of a limb, deafness, fearful of being along, etc.

Name of client's GP

Is the client aware that you have referred them to the EPIC Project?

Please return this form to:
THE EPIC PROJECT – STIRLING ROYAL INFIRMARY
(Tel 73151 ext 43961)

Tick the box which applies

1. Does the older person live alone or with others

The older person lives alone	□
The older person lives with others	□

Marital status of older person (tick as appropriate)

Widow/widower	□
Never married	□
Single parent	□
Divorced/separated	□
Spouse/partner in residential or other longterm care	□
Don't know status	□

Tick with whom

Spouse/partner	□
Family or friends	□
Other/don't know	□

Now answer the following question by circling the appropriate response:

	Answer			Answer about others living in the household		
2. Is the older person unable to get about outdoors on his/her own (even using a stick, zimmer or other aid)?	YES	NO	DK			
3. Does the older person have a history of falls or a well founded fear of falling?	YES	NO	DK			
4. a) Is the older person forgetful about things?	YES	NO	DK			
b) If YES to 4a, does this put him/her or other at risk?	YES	NO	DK			
5. Do you think the older person has problems with incontinence?	YES	NO	DK			
6. Is the older person failing to take care of themself in important ways such as failing to eat adequately, failing to keep the house warm enough, and/or neglecting their appearance?	YES	NO	DK			
7. Does the older person need more help at times during the day, evening or night (even if already receiving some assistance from family, friends/neighbours, or social and/or health agencies)?	YES	NO	DK			
8. If there is a relative or friend who makes a substantial contribution to care is this person under physical or emotional strain?	YES	NO	DK			
9. Has the older person had any of the following occurrences within the last two years?						
a) Lost somebody s/he cared about through death, moving or placement in residential or other longterm care?	YES	NO	DK	YES	NO	DK
b) Been hospitalised?	YES	NO	DK	YES	NO	DK
c) Only ask for those living with others Given up his/her own home and moved in with family, friends or others	YES	NO	DK	YES	NO	DK
10. Only ask for those living alone Is the older person without anyone living nearby, on whom they can rely/call for help in an emergency?	YES	NO	DK	YES	NO	DK

Appendix 8.2: After Care Plan

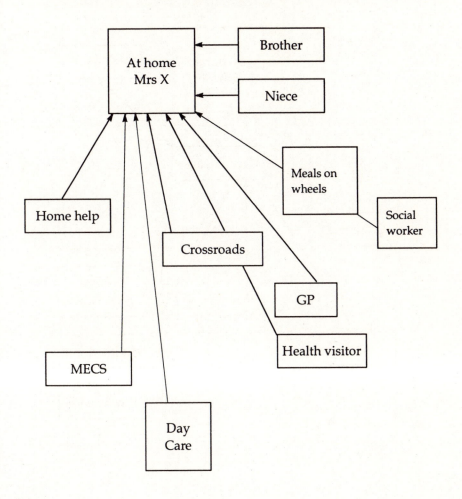

Appendix 8.3: After Care Plan

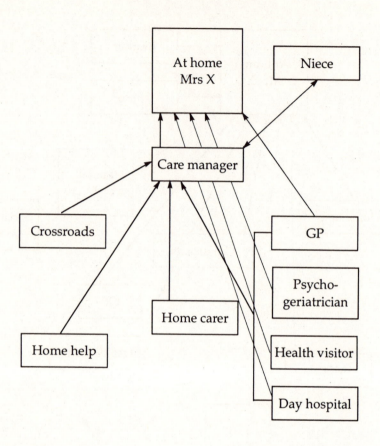

POINTS FOR DISCUSSION

1. Discuss how each of the components of care management have particular application to working with people with dementia and their carers.

2. Consider the aims and setting for care management in the EPIC Project. What are the main lessons to be learnt?

3. According to the SSI and SWSG guidelines, assessment is one of six core tasks that make up the process of care management. Discuss the relevance of each of the tasks for working with people with dementia and their carers, namely:

   (i) Publishing information

   (ii) Determining the level of assessment

   (iii) Assessing need

   (iv) Care planning

   (v) Implementing the care plan

   (vi) Monitoring and review

CHAPTER NINE

New Skills for Social Workers

Mary Marshall, Jan Stringer, Anne Marie Wright

The first part of this final chapter is a case study about a man with Downs's syndrome and Alzheimer's disease. It was chosen to make the point that there are constant new challenges even within the field of dementia. The second part reflects more generally on the issues raised with implications for further new skills needed in social work with reference to people with dementia which have not yet been fully addressed.

CASE STUDY

Most people with Down's syndrome will get Alzheimer's disease in late middle age, but this has not been an issue until recently, now that people with Down's syndrome live longer than ever before. There are very complex issues for social workers arising out of new groups of people like these, not least because the way we organise our services does not accommodate them.

The case study is in three parts. In the first Jan Stringer, the social worker, describes the work of the various social workers with John until he started attending the day centre for people with dementia. Then Anne Marie Wright, the day centre organiser, gives an account of the way the day centre approached involving John. In the third section, Jan Stringer brings the story of John up to date.

> John was born in 1924 with Down's syndrome. He lived a very sheltered life with his parents until his mother died in 1974, and his father never accepted his disability. He had two older married sisters and on the death of his mother went to live with one of them and her husband (Mr and Mrs B).
>
> At the age of fifty one he began attending an Adult Training Centre – his first experience of life outside the immediate family.

He remained at the ATC until he was sixty one when he 'retired'; the staff there felt that his needs had changed and that alternative day care resources should be sought. At this point he was allocated to an Area Social Work Team who worked towards finding him alternative day care and respite care at weekends to give support to Mr and Mrs B, both of which were now in their seventies.

A place was found at a local day centre for frail elderly people, and he built up to going there five days a week. However, given his short concentration span and agitated behaviour, the days began to get shortened. He continued at the day centre and spent weekends at a local hostel for people with a mental handicap for some two years, but during the latter stages concern was being expressed both about John's deterioration in health and that of his sister and brother-in-law, both of whom have arthritis with Mr B having a heart condition as well.

Reports and letters at this time referred to the fact that John had a persistent desire to go to the toilet and get undressed. He was also continually washing his hands. He frequently argued with other clients; touching them, poking his tongue out and threatening them with his fist. He was noted as being disruptive in groups, unable to understand that it was not always 'his turn'. It was recognised that he had 'a cheerful disposition at times, friendly and helpful, but from a management point of view every aspect of his care needs constant supervision'.

The hostel where he was receiving respite care noticed a rapid speeding up of his aging process and his sister became more and more anxious that she was not going to be able to offer him the same standards of care. John was reallocated to a social worker when it became clear that he was no longer going to be able to attend the day care centre. The respite care hostel felt that he ought to be placed in longterm Part IV accommodation (local authority home for older people).

The initial social work assessment and recommendation considered a Part IV placement would be appropriate and felt that he should be cared for in the same way as any other frail, forgetful elderly person. This was in line with the region's policy of 'normalisation', whereby an elderly client with learning difficulties requiring residential care could be placed in a residential resource for the elderly providing that they were 'Part IV fit'.

In October 1989 John was placed in a local authority Part IV home for the elderly. At a review held a month later his behaviour pattern was similar to that noted by the day centre and hostel; he appeared confused and disorientated, he was constantly changing his clothes and had a disturbed sleep pattern. He had been knocked over by another resident and had received verbal abuse from other residents. The staff there concluded that they felt that John was inappropriately placed, saying: 'We do not have the experience and staffing for John's needs and one-to-one relationship, therefore alternative care needs to be considered'.

The social work team assessed the situation in November, looked at possible alternatives and arrived at the following conclusions:

1. The original decision to place John within a Part IV setting was within regional policy. He had been assessed as 'Part IV fit' by a geriatrician.

2. He would be inappropriately placed within the local longstay hospital for people with learning difficulties and, in any case, they were in the process of discharging patients back into the community.

3. There were no vacancies in traditional longstay local authority hostels for people with learning disabilities. Upon enquiring they discovered that a number of existing residents in these hostels were elderly and themselves in need of Part IV accommodation.

4. John's sister and brother-in-law were no longer able to care for him, even on a temporary basis.

5. If the existing Part IV home could not cope, John would 'block' a respite bed.

6. If the local authority units could not cope, it was unlikely that a private unit would be able to do so.

7. John was not suited to a landlady scheme, or supported accommodation such as ARK housing.

It was therefore decided to request that extra staff be located at the Part IV home, for a limited period, whilst John and the other residents adjusted to their new circumstances. Complementary day care was considered at this stage but was felt to be inappropriate as it may have added to John's confusion.

At a case conference the following month the staff said that they were unable to offer him one-to-one attention, and that he appeared to spend his time walking 'aimlessly' around the unit. They thought that he was unhappy as he was constantly packing his bags in order to 'go home' and there was an increase in the number of times that he was throwing himself on the floor for attention. He had also been hit on the head with a slipper by another resident when he wandered into her room whilst she was asleep. The home requested that respite care at the hostel be increased.

The following March John was allocated to me as a longterm worker. Whilst pursuing an alternative longterm residential resource for John, I explored some day care resources. He commenced a 'social' group run by volunteers for older people with learning difficulties which met once a week and I arranged a two week respite holiday in B... John continued respite with the hostel, but this was being queried by their staff.

At this time he was assessed by a consultant psychiatrist specialising in learning difficulties, who noted his aggressive behaviour and the likelihood that he would begin to show signs of dementia. It was the opinion of the psychiatrist that John's problems were due to:

1. His learning difficulties and Down's syndrome.

2. The resistance on the part of other residents to accept him.

3. His previous very sheltered life with his carers.

It was felt that he was entitled to care in the community for as long as possible, as with any other elderly person, and small group living was recommended in supported accommodation for people with learning difficulties but for an 'elderly clientele'.

The situation over the next year clarified some of the problems but brought disappointments. John remained at the Part IV Home but the hostel withdrew the offer of respite care. They pointed out that it was unusual to offer respite care to a residential home, but they had done so as he was only there temporarily; but that was over a year ago, and they felt that being placed in two situations only added to John's confusion. Also, they needed the bed for their ongoing work of providing respite care for those who were remaining within the community.

John's provocative behaviour within the 'social' group had led to his placement with them reluctantly being withdrawn. The end result of all this was that the Part IV Home now found itself isolated in its care of John, whose needs had not altered in the sixteen months he had been with them. If anything, they had increased; and they pointed out that they felt that it was an inappropriate placement in the first place.

As the field social worker, I had approached the private and voluntary sector, re-explored local authority resources and local supported landladies. John's needs, particularly the level of supervision, excluded supported landladies, who do not employ night staff. The fundamental issue appeared to lie with John's age, as resources across the board appeared to have an age limit of about fifty five. Resources which extended this age range were struggling when dealing with residents with learning difficulties who had become elderly or frail and who possibly had dementia. They themselves were likely to be trying to refer their own clients to 'more appropriate resources'. I then began to consider the possibility of approaching resources available for those with dementia, and I contacted the coordinator of a local club which met once a week.

I had mixed feelings when John was assessed by a psychogeriatrician who confirmed that he may have dementia. That opened the door to other potential resources, but it seemed almost unjust that John required another 'label' in order to avail himself of resources which might meet his needs. My correspondence when referring to him would now read '... elderly Down's syndrome gentleman with possible dementia...'

The experience of a local resource –
The co-ordinator's view

When John's social worker first got in touch with me, it was to ask if I could accept a 64-year-old gentleman with Down's syndrome at our small day centre for people with dementia. My immediate and spontaneous reaction was 'Yes'; if he had dementia he should be as eligible as anyone else for a place. We had someone with Parkinson's Disease, a diabetic lady and a gentleman with a catheter in, so why not someone with Down's syndrome?

The main thing we had to have confirmed was that he did have some degree of dementia diagnosed, as that is a requirement for all those who do come to us. The other dilemma was that our group exists to provide respite care for carers in order for the individual to remain in their own home. When a person moves into permanent residential care the placement in our centre must cease (although we sometimes build bridges for six to eight weeks if that is helpful or appropriate). John, however, had not had his placement at the home confirmed, so it was community care for him (as opposed to mental handicap hospital) and in this case we would be providing respite for his carers at the Part IV Home, because of the special needs John had, until his permanent placement could be worked out.

Once it was confirmed that he had dementia, John was fully eligible for a place with us. However, in view of the antagonism towards him in the home from other residents, I felt that we needed to plan his coming to us as carefully as possible. I decided that we would first of all invite him to come and have lunch with us at the club, and then stay on for the remaining hour. This would enable us to watch for any adverse reaction from our members and also give us an idea of what he was like and how his social worker handled him. Our group was fairly used to visitors and I had carefully prepared them just before they came.

The lunch and afternoon went well and he shook everyone by the hand. With a one-to-one ratio of members/helpers we were able to watch reactions and none appeared adverse. So John joined us. Each member comes for a trial period of four weeks and John was the same. He settled in very well and the group warmed to him. As with all new members, it took us some weeks really to get to know him, to learn what his interests were, what he could or could not do and how to relate well to him as a person. This kind of assessment is done over a period of weeks with all members; we have eight, and all are individuals, all are different, with different interests and skills. John presented the same challenge to us as everyone else had done.

John's manners were excellent. Although very slow at meal times he was always most appreciative of all he was given and his 'That's good' was a great morale boost to those who prepared and served lunch. Hand washing was something of an obsession, and he often had sore, red hands; sometimes I felt that this was something that he did when he was bored, and as he became settled with us and was fully occupied, it virtually stopped. He never liked taking part in 'messy' activities though!

We try to have a good mixture of social/group activities, stimulation and restful activities, individual and creative activities; trying to concentrate on what skills people still have and not showing up what they can no longer do. We try to give everyone a sense of their own worth.

Our day begins at 9.30 am with tea and toast. It is a time of relaxing, chatting, informal reality orientation, sharing of news, looking at postcards people send us, and so on. Then comes some mental stimulation, usually in the form of a quiz. If this involved bean bags or balls, John would take his turn with everyone else and he got real pleasure from just being part of a group. If it was too complicated for him he would help with the washing up (as do all members) or help set the table or arrange the table flowers. After this time we usually broke up into small groups with a one-to-one ratio of helpers. John enjoyed painting or colouring, either free style or in his Mickey Mouse book (he was a great Mickey fan). We did not let him spend all his time on this as he did a lot in the home and we wanted to concentrate on other things at the club. He painted shells or plaster of Paris models which we made for him. He made rag pictures and did simple jigsaws. It was often difficult to get simple jigsaws which were not babyish. He could play dominoes and hold his own on an equal footing in any group.

He enjoyed looking at books of animals, royalty or film stars. We did not leave him alone with them but would talk to him about who or what he could see. He also enjoyed team games of beetle or skittles and because he could count and tell his colours he was able to do these on an equal basis with others, and often better! He joined with others in doing craft work and when one member made large pictures of Mickey and Minnie Mouse on thick card, painted them and punched holes on them, John was able to 'sew' them with brightly coloured laces; he loved doing that.

Before lunch each day we have a period of music and move-ment: he loved this activity and excelled in it. He had a deep rich voice and would often stand by the pianist and sing. Some after-noons we had a percussion group and his sense of music and rhythm made him far more able than the others. They recognised this and took great pleasure in his achievements.

Most months we have an outing. John loved going out to new places. Occasionally, as the minibus came to his home he would cry and say that he did not wish to 'go in there'. Whether this was real unhappiness or an emotional aspect of dementia was not easy to say.

On the whole the club found John much easier to handle than the home did, but there were several reasons for this:

1. We only had him for one day a week, and he was not with us during the evening when he was often at his most restless, refusing to go to bed or wandering into other people's rooms.

2. None of our members' personal possessions was threatened as everything belonged to the club, and all of us were on neutral territory.

3. There was no antagonism from the members; they seemed to be more tolerant of John, partly for the above reasons and partly due to good preparation by the helpers before he came and ongoing monitoring of reactions.

4. Our one-to-one ratio was a definite bonus. John's individual interests were catered for, he was stimulated, and he did not have time to be bored.

There were times when he needed firmness; for instance, when he went over to people and made animal noises, we needed to say firmly but kindly: 'John, please do not make that noise, you are not a pig/dog/cow'. We would immediately distract his attention and involve him in something else more interesting before he had time to be aggressive.

By late autumn, after he had been with us for about six months, his condition was beginning to deteriorate. He very suddenly seemed to become an 'old man'. He became more bald, began to walk with something of a shuffle, became more restless and less able to concentrate. It became more difficult to keep him 'interested' in things. His eyesight deteriorated as cataracts began to form. This, in common with many of our members, made it more difficult for him to see to do craft work or play games.

His sleep pattern was also becoming more disturbed and being up at night made him more drowsy during the day. He began to have more and more hallucinations which sometimes upset him and made him cry, or else, more commonly, made him hit out aggressively at whoever was sitting next to him, so we had to ensure that he was 'sandwiched' between two helpers. He was given sedation by the staff at the home, but this made him sleepy at the club, so we tried not to give him any unless he was really aggressive or restless. Instead we made up a small brown suitcase (rummage box) filled with bags of shells, coloured stones, marbles, model cars and so forth and we would sit with him and look through it.

Eventually things 'came together'. His placement was confirmed as permanent in the home and he was offered two days a week day care at the hospital with the possibility of a third in the future. By February, when he had been with us for almost a year, some of our other members had also began to deteriorate and become more difficult and we were finding it hard to cope. We were assured that he could get his extra day elsewhere if he no longer came to us.

We were all sad to lose him and miss him still. He brought much to the club through his presence and our members, without exception, warmed to him, felt 'sorry' for him and would try to 'mother' him at times. In a way it gave them more confidence in themselves because they knew that they were 'not like John'; they were better off, even if their memories were bad!

He fitted well into a dementia group and the length of stay was average or better than average as most members deteriorate and have to move on between six and nine months later. The structure of the day, the high member/helper ratio, the variety and length of activities made it a good setting for him. The challenge of John was, for us, no different from the rest of our members with dementia. We treated him with dignity, as an individual. There will be many more examples of 'John' in years to come. How well will they be catered for, and who will provide the services?

Final comments

The conclusion of John's situation was a degree of irony. Over a period of twenty months when he was considered 'Part IV fit', the expressed view was that he was inappropriately placed within Part IV accommodation. By November 1991 he was reassessed by a psychogeriatrician who concluded that was no longer 'Part Iv fit'. At a final case conference that November this information was shared with a number of agencies. The home seemed alarmed that, beyond themselves, who had cared for him for over two years on a 'temporary basis' his only future lay within a longterm hospital. The expressed staff view was that his remaining with them, despite the exigencies, was highly preferable to his placement in a longterm ward.

On November 28 1991 John's placement with a local authority home for the elderly became permanent, despite the fact that he was no longer 'Part IV fit!' In addition, to complement and support his care, the hospital offered day care twice a week and the potential for respite care. John has remained in residential care for the elderly.

Without exception the professional agencies and carers who had contact with John found him to be a kind gentleman with a warm personality. For the residential staff in the local authority home, their feelings for John influenced their approach. Contradictory discussions were common place, for example, 'We would not like to see him placed in a longterm hospital...'despite awareness that a non-institutional resource did not exist.

As his field social worker it was difficult not to be moved by John's spontaneity, warmth and sincerity which jarred with the knowledge that his future appeared to lie with a longterm hospital placement. Discussions were often laced with quite emotive feelings of despair, anxiety and frustration. Given that the regional resource situation remains the same, I have no doubt that at this moment a field social worker is also wrestling their way through similar predicaments for their client.

MORE GENERAL REFLECTIONS

There are going to be large numbers of people like John in the future because most people with Down's syndrome get dementia in late middle age. The reasons for this are not clear; it may be premature ageing or it may be a chromosomal link. There is no way of knowing what number this is likely to be since there are no figures about the numbers of people there are with Downs's syndrome by age. It is a worrying issue, because people with Down's syndrome are the most likely to be discharged from longstay hospitals into community facilities because they are often such pleasant, well mannered people. Very few facilities in the community are staffed to meet the needs of someone with dementia and there will soon be no longstay hospital beds. Other groups with early onset include a small proportion of people with AIDS, some people with chronic drinking problems and a few people with early Alzheimer's disease. These people with early onset dementia are not a large group but they all present very difficult and often very distressing problems to social workers.

John, like people from many new client groups, has needs which overlap different services or, perhaps more accurately, has needs which are not the responsibility of any service. Most of the newly emerging younger groups of people with dementia are in the same position. People with AIDS and dementia are often not appropriately cared for by AIDS services; people with alcohol-related dementia are often misplaced in adult psychiatry units. Younger people with Alzheimer's disease fit neither the adult psychiatry services nor the psychogeriatric service.

Ideally, we need new services for these groups of people, but their numbers are not yet great enough to have put sufficient pressure on the system. Also, we have the fall-back service of the big psychiatric hospitals at the moment, but not for much longer. Smaller, and more appropriate, local services are going to be required soon.

SERVICE DEVELOPMENT

This raises the issue of service development skills for which there was not space for a separate chapter in this book. These are underdeveloped in social work literature but they will have to be learned and recorded as the new community care arrangements settle down. We are going to have to get very good at identifying a need and translating this into an appropriate service which we then set up. John's social workers saw her job as manoevering within a set of unsuitable services, each with its own criteria and rationing systems. The label attached to the client was clearly of greatest importance. Each service had disadvantages and one is left with the impression that it was the least bad, rather than the best, service which was the aim.

This model of social work may be a thing of the past as we move towards needs-led, smaller, local services or packages of care. What John needed was a unit near his relatives which provided individual care and which adapted to his diminishing competence as his dementia progressed: a tall order. Adult placement may be the answer for some people like John, properly supported by respite and other places to go during the day. Alternatively, as the numbers of people like John increase, it may be possible to staff some of the group living units for people with learning disability in such a way that extra care is provided over time. Social workers are going to be part of numerous experiments over the next few years which cannot fail to be more appropriate if the needs-led ethos is allowed to prevail. Service development requires vision, entrepreneurial skills, determination and patience as well as the skills of identifying needs and translating them into a service.

John's social worker is clearly preoccupied with finding him somewhere to live. Whether or not she had used her skills of direct work with people with dementia and their carers is not clear. What is clear is that she was an extraordinarily determined and energetic social worker with a real commitment to doing her very best for this man. One suspects that she used her direct skills all the time in helping the staff to cope with John at the residential home and in the various day settings he attended, in counselling the relatives and in helping John himself to make the best of the opportunities he was offered.

GROUP CARE

It is in group care settings that a great deal of the intensive work with individuals takes place. This day centre demonstrates exemplary practice in its focus on the individual rather than the label, although the correct diagnosis at the outset is the key to a place. The day centre used the strengths of the group in the care of the individual. One of the inspiring characteristics of this account is the implication that a day centre full of people with dementia uses them as a resource for one of their members: they like to care for John. The account also describes how the volunteers approached John's needs in a planned fashion, adapting their roles as his disease progressed. There are many lessons here about working with volunteers which probably deserve a chapter of their own.

The chapter on counselling was written by a fieldworker in Australia. In the UK, where going somewhere for counselling is less common, much of the therapeutic work with people with dementia takes place in longstay settings. Validation therapy, for example, which is about exquisite listening to people with dementia and learning to communicate symbolically and emotionally, although rare, is more common in day and residential settings. Similarly, we have concentrated in this book on groupwork in the field, but most of the groupwork with people with dementia takes place in day and longstay settings. It is not surprising that most of the groups in the chapter on groupwork were in some way attached to a group care setting.

Although raised in the first chapter, the skills of supporting and assisting care staff who are providing the group care a lot of our clients need, do not have a chapter of their own because so little is known about them. Clearly to do this effectively we need to have some idea about the tasks of group care and the inevitable tension between providing for the individual and the group. We also have to realise that caring for the staff is fundamental if they are to have the personal resources they need to do the job. Both the case study and the chapter on using the past provide some pointers. Using the past takes the novel approach of asking the staff who they find most difficult and then concentrating on them. The success of this intervention was as much about motivating the staff as about the model of care being tried. Staff will have felt that an outside social worker was acknowledging the extreme problems they have with some residents, was offering a possible approach and was giving them lots of strokes for trying.

NEW SKILLS FOR THE FUTURE

In choosing the chapters of this book we had to decide what were the most important new skills to include and which ones to leave out. So far I have mentioned that we left out the new groups of people with dementia. We left out the negotiating and manoevering skills and we left out the staff support skills, except by implication. We also left out particular areas of work such as meeting the sexual needs of people with dementia and coping with their sometimes difficult sexual behaviour. And we left out the issue of meeting the spiritual needs of people with dementia. These last two gaps are being recognised by workers in the field but we will need to accumulate a literature and more experience before we can write them up. We have chosen relatively well established skills for this book and ones where there is a literature and there is experience even if it is with other client groups.

We decided that the most fundamental skills were the direct skills, where social workers themselves work with people with dementia and their carers. Only the chapter on care management covers the indirect skills of service organisation to any extent. It is our view that indirect skills have to be built onto a competence with the direct ones. In our view Jan Stringer could not have done such an excellent job for John unless she had been able to work directly with John and the relatives. We do not know if she had basic groupwork skills with clients; she did not require to take them out of her tool kit for this particular man, although she will undoubtedly have had to use general groupwork skills in the numerous case conferences and meetings she attended to negotiate help for him.

One of the troubles is that, as social workers, on the whole, we do not give enough attention to these very basic skills, so we decided to cover them explicitly. We ought all to be able to counsel, to run an effective group and to work with families. We wanted to avoid being too basic so we chose social workers to write for us who had experience and strong views about particular approaches. Thus we describe a systemic approach to family work which may not suit everyone but which emphasises the need for a family approach. We chose a model of empowerment around training but the principle of working in a way which empowers our clients does not depend on what we are doing with them: it is about treating people in a way which recognises their strengths and expertise.

Another gap is advocacy skills. Clearly Jan Stringer is using them in her work with John. There are very few advocacy schemes as such with people with dementia. There is an urgent need for social workers to draw together the skills of advocacy in relation to people with dementia. It probably requires us to be more explicit about the skills of communication with people with dementia. It will not be long before we know much more about these with the current pressure to obtain the users' view of services and this includes users with dementia.

Another major gap is to work with people from ethnic minorities. This has been staggeringly neglected. Dementia services seldom think about ethnic minorities and ethnic minority services seldom explicitly address the needs of their users who have dementia. There is at the moment very little expertise to draw on in both advocacy and work with ethnic minorities, although both are beginning to receive more attention.

A third, and less obvious gap in the experience of social workers is around death. How do we ensure a dignified death for people with dementia? How do we talk about death to people with dementia? There is some expertise in working with carers as their relative approaches death and in bereavement but this needs to be filled out from the perspective of the person with dementia.

The common thread that links many of the gaps in our expertise is the face-to-face work with people with dementia. We have tried to include it wherever possible in the book. The reality of the last ten years, as services and skills have developed, is that we have concentrated primarily on carers. There are a lot of good reasons for this. Their needs are more obvious, the priority of supporting them as the main resource is unquestionable, we can communicate with carers.

CONCLUSION

It is our hope that this book has built on what social workers reading it already know and has at the same time given some idea about why we are so enthusiastic about social work in this field. It is very exciting to work in a field which is changing all the time; where new skills are emerging and new knowledge is underpinning them. There is still a long way to go. A priority is for social workers with expertise to write it up to supplement the meagre resources at present available. Another is to fight for opportunities to experiment with new skills. Family therapy, for example, ought to be widespread, because this is so often a family issue that puts overwhelming strain on dysfunctional families. The current changes to the way that social services are delivered should teach us many things about the particular needs of people with dementia and their carers and new ways of meeting them. We live in exciting times, and ones which are potentially going to do a great deal to improve the lives of people with dementia and their carers.

Contributors

Alan Chapman is the Training Officer for the Dementia Services Development Centre at the University of Stirling.

J. Crawford was the Project Leader of the EPIC care management project funded by Central Regional Council Social Work Department and Forth Valley Health Board.

Iain Gardner was responsible for establishing the Counselling and Advisory Service at the Alzheimer's Society of Victoria in Australia. He now lectures in Management And Organisational Behaviour at University of Melbourne.

Faith Gibson is a Reader in Social Work at the University of Ulster at Jordanstown, N. Ireland.

Mary Marshall is the Director of the Dementia Services Development Centre at the University of Stirling.

Katrina Myers is the Training Officer (elderly) for Central Regional Council Social Work Department.

Philip Seed is Honorary Lecturer at the University of Dundee, Department of Social Work where he was, until his recent retirement, Senior Research Fellow. He is also Chairman of Raddery Residential Special School for emotionally damaged children.

Joanne Sherlock was a counsellor with the Counselling and Advisory Service at the Alzheimer's Society of Victoria in Australia. She is currently a member of a Regional Aged Care Assessment Team associated with a regional aged care facility in Melbourne.

Jan Stringer was a generic field social worker for Lothian Regional Council Social Work Department when she wrote the case study.

Anne Marie Wright is the organiser of the Holy Corner Tuesday Club, Edinburgh.

Index

Abuse 72
Activities 102–4, 106, 108–9, 118, 156–7, 159
Admission 85
Advocacy 7, 16, 78, 80, 110, 112, 137, 142, 163–4
Aging 151, 160
Alzheimer's Disease Society/Alzheimer's Scotland 6, 84
Anxiety 9–10, 41, 134, 140
Assessed 154
Assessment 5, 13, 18–20, 26, 28, 33, 35–6, 42, 49, 69–73, 76, 85, 114, 125–149, 151, 156
Assessor 135–7
Attention seeking 153

Behaviour(s) 3, 5, 8–10, 12–3, 24, 27, 29, 31, 36, 38, 45, 48, 50, 53–4, 65, 68, 73, 75–6, 80, 83–4, 86, 88–9, 92–3, 100, 119, 152–3
Bereavement 84, 164
British Association of Social Workers 84
Burnout 89

Care in Community 113–4, 119–20, 130, 142, 153
Care plan 50, 85, 125, 128, 135, 137–8, 140–2
Care Management 2, 125–144, 149, 163
Care Manager 126–31, 133–35, 137, 139–41, 143
Carer(s) 1, 3, 5–8, 11, 13, 17, 28–30, 33–35, 42–3, 45, 57–8, 60, 69–70, 76–7, 81–5, 87–98, 100, 106–7, 112, 115–22, 125–9, 132–8, 140–3, 153, 155, 163–5
Carers National Association 6
Case Finding 131
Challis & Davis 131
Choice(s) 77, 110, 115, 117, 122, 129–30, 134, 139
Client centred 77
Community Care 1, 6, 12, 45, 54, 125, 130, 161
Conflict 12–3, 64, 67–8, 78, 126
Consumer 110, 138
Contracts 23, 71–2, 76, 80, 112
Control 116, 118, 122
Counselling 1–2, 16–39, 63, 85, 114, 116, 137, 161–2
Counsellor 20–3

Crisis 27, 36, 68, 71, 95, 132
Crossroads 100, 129, 132, 139–40

Day hospital 89, 91, 106
Day centre 85, 107, 109, 150, 162
Day care 13, 55–6, 58, 92, 115, 153, 159
Death 21, 30, 86, 164
Dependency 111
Depression 4, 26, 67–8
Disorientated 86, 114, 125
Disorientation 137, 152
Down's Syndrome 150–160
Driving 76
Drugs 106

Early onset 92–3
Empathy 137
Empowerment 2, 110–124, 130, 163
Ethnic 78, 79, 164
Evaluation 23, 76, 86

Family assessment wheel 69, 71, 80
Family(ies) 2, 11, 14, 16, 18–20, 24, 26, 28–9, 34, 37, 54, 56, 58, 60, 63–5, 67–73, 75–80, 82–3, 88–9, 100–1, 164

Gender 77
Generic 77
Genogram(s) 73, 75, 80
Graduate carer 89
Grandparent(s) 73–4